D1460535

CARING
FOR THE SICK

CARING
FOR THE SICK

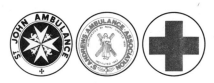

Authorised by
St. John Ambulance
St. Andrew's Ambulance Association
The British Red Cross Society

1982

Trade edition first published in Great Britain in 1982 by
Dorling Kindersley Limited, 9 Henrietta Street,
Covent Garden, London WC2E 8PS

British Library Cataloguing in Publication Data
Caring for the sick.
1. Home care services
I. St. John Ambulance
II. St. Andrew's Ambulance Association
III. British Red Cross
362.1'4   RA645.3
ISBN 0-86318-002-7
ISBN 0-86318-003-5 Pbk
ISBN 0-86318-008-6 Counterpack

Printed in Italy by A. Mondadori, Verona

CONTENTS

INTRODUCTION 8

THE PATIENT'S SURROUNDINGS: Helping the patient to avoid the dangers of the environment **17**

Planning the patient's room **18**   Planning a child's room **20**

COMFORT AND MOBILITY: Helping the patient to move and maintain a comfortable position **23**

Bedmaking **24**   Moving the patient **32**
Pressure areas **29**   Aids to walking **37**
Positions for bedrest **30**   The patient in a wheelchair **38**
Aids to comfort in bed **31**

WASHING AND BATHING: Helping the patient to keep his body clean **39**

Bathing **40**   Caring for the eyes **45**
Aids to bathing **41**   Caring for the mouth **46**
Giving a bed bath **43**   Caring for the hair **47**
Shaving and washing **44**   Bathing the new baby **48**
Caring for the nails **45**

CLOTHING: Helping the patient to dress and undress and to select clothing **49**

Dressing and undressing **50**   Clothing for the incontinent **54**
Aids to dressing **51**   Dressing the new baby **55**
Selecting clothing **52**   Selecting children's clothing **56**

EATING AND DRINKING: Helping the patient to take an adequate diet and feed himself **57**

The importance of a balanced diet **58**   The helpless patient **63**
Types of diet **59**   The unconscious patient **63**
Categories of nutrient **60**   Aids to eating and drinking **64**
Food habits **62**   Minor digestive problems **66**
The patient who can feed himself **62**   Breast-feeding **67**
The blind patient **63**   Bottle-feeding **69**
The patient without teeth **63**

GIVING MEDICINES: Helping the patient to take and care for his medicines **71**

Medicines by mouth **72**   Administering drops **74**
Drugs by rectum **73**   Care and custody of medicines **75**
Drugs by inhalation **73**   Giving medicines to children **76**
Drugs by injection **73**

ELIMINATION: Helping the patient to deal with his excretions   **77**

Basic care	78	Incontinence	84
Aids in the lavatory	79	Aids for incontinence	86
Urine	80	The patient with a stoma	88
Faeces	82	Changing the new baby	90

REST AND SLEEP: Helping the patient to relax and maintain good
sleeping habits   **93**

Causes of wakefulness	94	The sick child	98
The new baby	97		

CONTROLLING TEMPERATURE: Helping the patient to maintain normal
body temperature   **99**

Hypothermia	100	Taking the respiratory rate	105
Aids to warmth	102	Inflammation	106
Fever	103	Applying local heat	107
Taking the temperature	104	Communicable diseases	108
Taking the pulse	105	Incubation and isolation periods	110

CARING FOR A WOUND: Helping the patient with an injury   **113**

How a wound heals	114	Applying a bandage	120
Preventing infection	114	Bandaging patterns	121
Sterilizing equipment	115	Making a triangular bandage	122
Using an aseptic technique	116	Applying a sling	122
Securing a dressing	118		

BREATHING DIFFICULTIES: Helping the patient to breathe more easily   **123**

Clearing a blocked nose	125	Giving oxygen	128
Controlling the cough	126	Oxygen for use in the home	129
Relieving spasm	126	Caring for a tracheostomy	130
Helping the breathless patient	127		

COMMUNICATION: Helping the patient to communicate his needs effectively   **131**

Non-verbal communication	132	The blind patient	134
Verbal communication	133	The non-English speaking patient	135
The patient who cannot talk	133	The confused patient	135
The deaf patient	134	Helping the mentally ill	136

RECOVERY AND REHABILITATION: Helping the patient towards
complete recovery   **137**

Patients newly discharged from hospital	138	Attendance at day centres	141
Day patients	140	Outpatients	142

RECREATIONAL ACTIVITIES: Helping the patient to make good use of his time   **143**

Stages of illness	**144**	Planning activities for children	**146**
Activities for the convalescent	**145**		

LEARNING AND RE-LEARNING: Helping the patient to overcome disabilities and master new skills   **147**

Difficulties with learning	**148**	The need to modify skills	**150**
The need to re-learn	**149**		

THE PATIENT WHO IS DYING: Helping the patient to a peaceful and dignified death   **151**

Feelings and fears about death	**152**	Different religious beliefs	**155**
Stages of grief	**152**	Helping the relatives	**155**
Making the patient comfortable	**153**	Practical help	**155**
The signs of approaching death	**154**		

USEFUL READING   156

USEFUL ADDRESSES   157

CONVERSION TABLES   158

INDEX   159

NOTES   164

ACKNOWLEDGMENTS   176

INTRODUCTION

Before you undertake to give nursing care you should first ask yourself: what is nursing? It *could* be defined merely as a set of tasks to be carried out in the shortest possible time, without considering individual likes or wants. In reality, nursing is the act of looking after an individual, helping him to do what he would do by himself if he could, and helping him in such a way that he does not lose his dignity and is encouraged to regain whatever independence he can as soon as he can.

The Needs of the Patient

The patient has the same needs as the person who is well. As you may have to help him do things that he cannot do for himself, you should know what the individual's basic needs are. Everyone needs:
- to be in a safe environment
- to move and maintain a comfortable position
- to keep his body clean and well-groomed and protect his skin
- to select suitable clothing and dress and undress
- to eat and drink adequately
- to eliminate
- to sleep and rest
- to maintain normal body temperature
- to breathe normally
- to communicate with others and express emotions, needs and fears
- to work at something that provides a sense of accomplishment
- to play or participate in various forms of recreation
- to learn, discover or satisfy the curiosity that is part of normal development and health
- to worship according to his faith.

Each of these needs should be considered in relation to the individual patient and you should ask yourself certain questions:
- what can the patient do unaided?

- is his present disability temporary or permanent?
- can he be taught or re-taught to do the things he is unable to do at present and so gain independence?
- if he cannot gain independence, can his family or friends help and, if so, will they require instruction?
- is professional help necessary through members of the health or social work teams?

If you try and answer these questions for yourself, you will be learning a great deal about the individual patient's needs. In planning individual care you must then do all you can to ensure that the physical, psychological, social, financial and spiritual needs of the individual are met.

Physical Needs

Physical needs include: being able to breathe, to eat and drink, to rest and sleep and to be safe in a stable environment. As you plan a daily routine for the patient you take account of these needs. You make sure he is washed, fed, gets enough sleep and stays secure in familiar surroundings. If the patient has to enter hospital, he may find that environment unfamiliar and unsettling, even hostile, in which case you need to do as much as you can to make him feel comfortable and at ease.

Psychological Needs

Basic psychological needs include: the need to be esteemed; the need to be valued, accepted and recognized as an individual; and the need for security and privacy. You can help to maintain the patient's self-esteem by encouraging as much independence as possible and by using a proper name and title. Many an elderly spinster feels annoyed and humiliated by being referred to as "gran". Take into account the patient's age, background, physical and mental condition and, depending on how well you know him, adjust your approach accordingly.

Ensure that privacy is available whenever the patient requires it, particularly if you are attending to his personal needs or if he wishes to talk quietly with a friend, lawyer or priest. Be alert to his feelings of insecurity, particularly if his illness has lasted for a long time and has left him severely incapacitated. Apprehension, fear and depression are often experienced by ill people.

Listen attentively to what the patient is saying; never appear hurried. Try instead to make him feel that you really care about him as a person. This is less difficult in the home than it is in a hospital or institution, where many patients are seeking your help and attention at the same time.

Young physically handicapped men and women often have sexual problems. Do not ask them questions, but if someone spontaneously confides in you let the doctor know what has been said. Psycho-sexual counselling may help not only them but their family also and the specialists in this field are very skilled people.

Social Needs

Whether young or old, the patient needs companionship. Visitors are always welcome, yet they can tire the patient. Try and assess the patient's condition to decide how much visiting is advisable and discuss your opinion with the family.

Radio or television can provide companionship but sets should be placed where they can be seen easily, heard without difficulty and switched off when not required. Turning off a television set some distance away can pose a problem: a set with remote control may be the answer. Alternatively, you should make sure that you are frequently available to respond to the patient's needs.

Children confined to bed for a long period may need to continue their education. Encourage parents to consult the head teacher of the child's school as he will give advice and can make any necessary arrangements.

Financial Needs

Many patients are worried about money and do not realize that they may be entitled to certain pensions or allowances. The district nursing sister can give advice or you can consult the local social security office or Citizens Advice Bureau.

Spiritual Needs

Whatever the patient's beliefs, they should be respected. If he would like to talk to his minister, priest or rabbi, a visit should be arranged. Make sure there is quiet and privacy during the visit and at any time when the patient would like to meditate or pray.

You should be aware of two other possibilities. The patient may have no religious belief; in this case he should not be embarrassed or made to feel ashamed. Alternatively, your beliefs may not be the same as his; under no circumstances should you try and force your ideas upon him.

The Role of the Volunteer

In this country there has been a long tradition of voluntary effort aimed at helping those in need, while the extra pressures on the National Health Service in recent years have led to increased emphasis being placed on the work of the voluntary organizations.

The Voluntary Organizations

Today the voluntary organizations play a vital part in assisting with, and extending the work of, the statutory organizations. Several categories of patient benefit particularly from their care.

Pressure on National Health Service beds has led to early discharge of patients from hospital into the community, or to people undergoing minor investigations as out-patients rather than in-patients. As family patterns change more and more elderly people

The Voluntary Aid Societies

The British Red Cross Society

The British Red Cross is an independent, paramedical organization. In peace-time Britain the Society trains its members, and members of the public, in first aid, nursing and associated subjects. Its voluntary, unpaid members work to alleviate suffering among the sick, the injured, the handicapped and the frail elderly. To train its members and maintain its services it relies on donations from the public.

The Society operates through local offices in England, Wales, Scotland, Northern Ireland, the Channel Islands, the Isle of Man and Britain's remaining colonies and dependencies. The pictures show the uniform members wear for nursing duties.

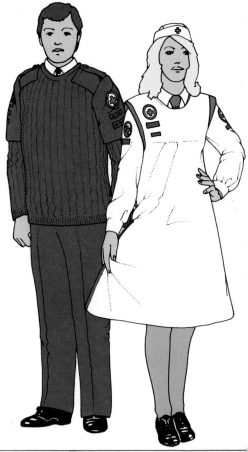

St. Andrew's Ambulance Association

1882 was the first year of activity for the St. Andrew's Ambulance Association, and 173 cases of accident and sudden illness were removed from the streets of Glasgow and taken to hospital by litter.

The Glasgow of Queen Victoria's reign was a rich, rapidly expanding industrial city. There was already a traffic problem, and the rapid increase in the number of road accidents was a matter of grave concern to a small handful of city doctors, while the industrial expansion and the advent of modern machinery were taking their own toll of life and limb. Before the year 1882

was much older, 500 members of the Association had been instructed "in the preliminary care and attention to meet the first needs of sufferers from accidents and bodily injuries and mutilation". That same year the Association provided itself with *one* ambulance — the first in Scotland.

Today, one hundred years later, the organization has no fewer than 230 different Sections with a total strength of 6000, plus 2000 Cadets, in addition to 20,000 Association members. The activities of the Association cover a wide range of humanitarian work, including in its teaching a knowledge

The St. John Ambulance

The Order of St. John of Jerusalem can be traced back to times before the Great Crusades, when the brothers tended pilgrims on their way to Jerusalem. Today it still has three great Foundations: the Opthalmic Hospital in Jerusalem, the Association which is responsible for training and the Brigade whose uniforms are so familiar at public functions. The local unit of the Brigade is the Division; here the members meet together each week to undergo training in first aid and nursing. Doctors and nurses who are also members of the Brigade meet with them to teach and supervise their practice. In any one year the Brigade carries out more than three million hours of duties. The pictures show the uniform members wear for nursing duties, at home or in hospital.

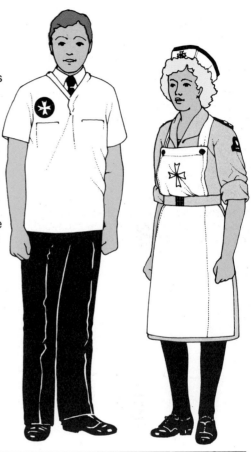

of first aid, nursing and allied subjects, distributed widely among all age groups of the public — from school-children to industrial and commercial concerns.

Classes are organized, followed by examinations, and successful candidates receive a Certificate of Proficiency. Competitions are arranged, while the Association also publishes textbooks, and organizes first aid films and visual aids.

The practical service is provided by uniformed and trained volunteers who carry out many voluntary duties throughout Scotland and are known as St. Andrew's Ambulance Corps. Trained first aid personnel are provided at all types of public function. Another feature of the service is the outings arranged for elderly people, blind people and physically handicapped children; trained men and/or women are also provided to accompany invalids or injured persons on journeys by land, air or sea, and there is a Medical Aids Service.

St. Andrew's Ambulance Association Cadet Corps has a strength of around 2000 boys and girls aged between 11 and 15, who are trained for service in the adult Sections.

are living on their own — these are people who often need help when they are well, let alone when they are ill. Many handicapped people live longer than used to be the case with the help of modern drugs, but require constant attention. The scope for voluntary effort is endless and the range of work carried out by the volunteer is extremely wide. Much is the extension of "good neighbourliness"; some is more organized and linked with professional workers such as the district nursing sister or social worker.

In the early 1960s a recognition of the importance of the volunteers' contribution led to the appointment of two Voluntary Service Organizers in the hospital service. Their task was to identify areas where volunteers could play a useful part and to recruit and place individuals where needed. Appointments of this kind have increased and Voluntary Service Organizers are now to be found in hospitals and in the Social Service Departments of local authorities.

The Individual Volunteer

This book is primarily intended for members of the voluntary aid societies but will also be of use to those who choose or need to give nursing care at home. As a volunteer you hold a unique place in society. When you give nursing care you are accepted by the patient, his relatives and friends, and by the professional workers in the health care team. You are expected to have certain qualities: you should be energetic, imaginative, independent, able to work alone or as part of a team, always willing, always reliable and always self-controlled. You should use tact and discretion; you should show sincerity, sympathy and understanding. You also need special skills: you should be gentle and dextrous, observant, reassuring, resourceful, able to communicate easily and to give explicit instructions.

You should always look neat and tidy, as this can inspire confidence in the patient and his family. Your hair should be kept controlled and your nails short

and clean. Shoes should be carefully chosen to
provide support and to remain silent as you move
around the sickroom. Many people smoke, but the
smell of smoke on the breath may be nauseating to
an ill person. You should also take care not to give
offence from body odour. If you are careful about
your own cleanliness and freshness you are more
likely to care about your patient's personal
appearance.

The Volunteer –
Patient Relationship

When someone is ill he becomes a patient. He will
probably feel insecure and need the support of
those around him. By going about your work in a
quiet and confident manner you can quickly gain the
respect and trust of the patient and his relatives. A
good question to ask is: "How would I like to be
cared for if I were ill?" If you can satisfy yourself
then you will satisfy the patient. Remember that
everyone has different likes and dislikes, so
whenever possible involve the patient in the
decisions that you make about his care.
   Maintaining a good volunteer-patient relationship
takes time as well as effort, but that is what nursing
is: time, effort and skill in the service of others.
   In the course of your work you may learn a great
deal about a patient. It is essential to remember that
information given to you by the patient or about the
patient should only be discussed with the doctor,
nurse or others professionally concerned with the
care of the patient. What is said and done in the
sickroom is not a subject for general comment or
conversation outside it. Any instructions given by
the doctor or professional nurse must be carried out
punctually and carefully. There must be loyalty to
the doctor and nurse at all times. If you observe these
rules you will find that your relationship with those
offering professional care is one of trust.

The Volunteer – Professional Relationship

The professional members of the health team are responsible for the patient. As a volunteer, you are only there to assist them. It is essential that you recognize your own limitations and at no time try and exceed them. You should never make decisions or undertake treatment without prior consultation. You must recognize that you are privileged in being accepted as part of the caring team and you should be prepared in all things to put the patient first.

Reliability is a key element in your relations with doctors and professional nurses. If you undertake a ward duty you should expect to fulfil it on a regular basis; otherwise the ward sister cannot plan the use of your experience and may be irritated at the waste of her valuable time. You should be prepared to give a commitment to training and keeping your skills up to date. If you do, you will find the professional nurse only too willing to help you gain the knowledge and the skill you need.

Several sections in this book are concerned with the general care of babies and children. Although not strictly speaking about nursing sick patients, it is felt that such information is relevant and important enough to be included here. The mother just discharged from hospital with her new baby, for instance, and all those offering her help could well benefit from some basic everyday information about looking after a newborn baby. A few points about safety and health — such as how to store medicines in the home or what sort of shoes a child should wear — will be found in the appropriate chapters.

For people whose main interest is in the information about children and babies, pages dealing exclusively with these subjects have been picked out by a blue border running around the edge of the page. It is hoped that in this way the information will be easy to find and use.

THE PATIENT'S SURROUNDINGS:
Helping the patient to avoid the dangers of the environment

THE PATIENT'S SURROUNDINGS

Healthy people are usually able to choose their environment. If anything makes it uncomfortable or dangerous, they are free to make adjustments or move away. The patient, however, is dependent upon those nursing him to see that his surroundings are safe.

As a volunteer, you may be asked to provide a safe environment for the patient. When people are ill their movement is usually restricted. They may be confined to bed in their own home or in hospital. Their physical surroundings matter greatly and

the bedroom and furniture should be selected with care. The general atmosphere in the room is also crucial. Family, friends, doctors and nurses all help to create it and their attitude largely determines whether or not the patient feels a burden. Always try and create a pleasant and cheerful atmosphere. Let the patient feel you have time to meet his every need. Be conscious of the privilege you have in serving the sick. Your forethought will give comfort to the patient as well as support to his family.

Planning the Patient's Room

The room in which the patient is nursed should be clean. The air can carry germs from one person to another and any dust stirred up can settle on food or a wound and so infect the patient. The room should also be free from unpleasant smells. Use an aerosol to disperse the smells of food, bedpans and any other unpleasant odours. Even flower-water smells if it is not fresh. The sense of smell is intensified in sickness, so this is important.

The room should be comfortably warm and well ventilated. If it is too hot, the patient may sweat and become uncomfortable; if it is too cold, he may chill. In winter additional heating will probably be necessary. Beware of draughts. An open fire increases ventilation, but it should be well guarded so that when the patient is out of bed there is no danger of his dressing gown catching fire. Smoking in bed is also dangerous, particularly if the patient is elderly or drowsy. Always provide a large ashtray that will not spill easily and try and stay with the patient until he has finished smoking.

Most people prefer to stay in their own bedroom when they are ill. It may be more convenient for you to move a sick person downstairs or to a room nearer the bathroom but do this only for his real well-being, not merely for your convenience.

Whenever possible nurse the patient in a single bed with a firm but comfortable mattress. Try and leave plenty of space around the bed for ease of movement and the placement of any essential equipment.

If there is a pleasant garden or an interesting view, place the bed so that the patient can see out of the window. On the other hand, if the room can be overlooked, there must be blinds or curtains that can be closed for privacy. These are also useful for controlling the light.

It is a good idea to leave everything the patient may need within easy reach of the bed, otherwise he may overbalance and fall when stretching for something or when getting out of bed to reach something. If a small hand bell is available, this is an added safety measure. A good bedside light is necessary for both patient and nurse, over and above the main lighting.

Take care what is left on the bedside table of a confused patient. For instance, if you leave disinfectant in a sputum cup he may drink from it by mistake. Remove medicines, especially bottles of tablets, as he may repeat the dose, forgetting what he has already taken. Remove cigarettes and matches in case he sets the bed alight.

If the patient is able to use the bathroom you should ensure that the passageways are clear and that nothing has been left on

Cupboard space for storing nursing equipment is a valuable bonus in the sickroom.

The ideal bed in which to nurse the patient is a single bed with access to it on three sides and a clear path between the bed and the door.

A table provides an ideal working surface for nursing equipment.

A commode near the bed is useful for a patient who is unable or unwilling to go as far as the bathroom.

A table within easy reach of the bed should have on it everything that the patient might need, including a good bedside light and perhaps a small hand bell.

A comfortable armchair should provide good support for the patient's back when he is relaxing out of bed.

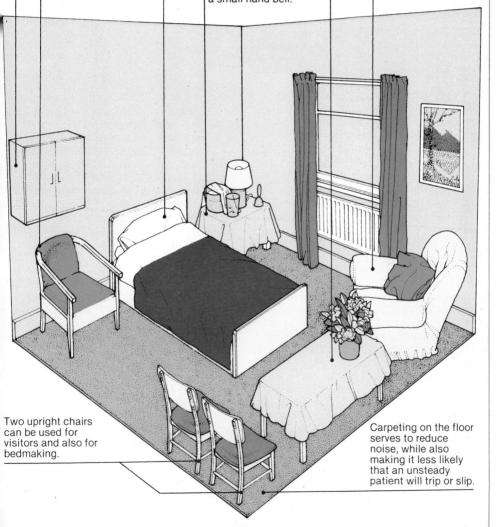

Two upright chairs can be used for visitors and also for bedmaking.

Carpeting on the floor serves to reduce noise, while also making it less likely that an unsteady patient will trip or slip.

the floor for him to trip over. Check also that the bathwater is not too hot and that there is a chair or stool in the bathroom.

Carpeting on the floor of the bedroom and tablecloths on the bedside table and work surfaces will help to reduce noise and at the same time protect the furniture. Be sensitive to noise: to an ill person every sound seems magnified. Noise can cause headache and make the patient irritable. You may need to turn down the radio and television or remove a ticking clock if it is disturbing him. Warn visitors to talk in a normal voice and not to shout: people often seem to think that because someone is ill he cannot hear.

Visitors, however welcome, can be exceedingly tiring. Try and restrict their number and the length of time they stay. This needs great tact and may tax your ingenuity if you are to control visitors without giving offence.

Selecting Furniture

If you are re-organizing a bedroom to make nursing easier, try and preserve the patient's feeling that it is still his room at home. Individual needs will vary, but certain minimum requirements usually apply to all sickrooms:
You should have:
● a firm table or locker for the patient within reach of the bed
● an armchair for the patient to sit in when he is allowed out of bed
● two chairs for bedmaking and for the use of visitors
● a commode if one is necessary and available
● a working surface for you: this should be protected by newspaper or plastic sheeting and covered with a clean paper towel
● cupboard space, useful if there are any dressings or equipment that the district nursing sister or midwife might use
● a clear pathway between the bed and the door, so that neither you nor the patient stumbles into the furniture in the dark.

Planning a Child's Room

The day of the formal nursery is past but, where possible, the new baby should have a room to himself, which in time can double as a playroom. The aim should be to provide a clean, airy room that is safe for its occupant. In the early months when the baby is confined to his cot there is little danger, but, once he begins to crawl, all sorts of hazards are to be found.

Parents usually decorate the room intended for the new baby: high gloss washable paint and vinyl papers are easily cleaned of grubby finger marks. A blackboard or an area of wall covered with formica gives the small child somewhere to draw and scribble as he wishes. The floor needs a covering as splinters from the wooden floor are dangerous when the child is crawling; linoleum or lino tiles are safe and colourful and many of the new synthetic materials are both soft and warm to the knees. If rugs are used, they should be bright, washable and, above all, non-slip. Curtains too should be washable and nursery prints are very attractive, but remember that pictures of witches and ogres may frighten small children.

Ventilation is important and should be achieved without draughts. As the child grows you should take care to see that he cannot fall from an open window. Lighting should be adequate, both for baby care in the early days and for the child to play by later on. Switches should be out of reach of small fingers and trailing flexes and unprotected sockets should also be made

A low chair without arms is ideal for breast-feeding a young baby.

Equipment for bathing the new baby is probably best kept in the bedroom until he is big enough to be bathed in the ordinary bath.

A drop-sided wooden cot is safe and will last for several years, until such time as the child is ready to move to an ordinary bed.

Adequate heating is essential for the new baby, especially at night. Central heating is probably the safest type of heating to have.

A surface for changing the baby's napkin is especially convenient if it is part of a unit containing storage space.

A floor covering of some sort is advisable, as a child learning to crawl and walk may get splinters in his skin from a wooden floor.

inaccessible. Toddlers will push things into electric sockets: it is essential to put a plug into an empty socket even if it is unconnected to any equipment.

Heating is essential, especially for the newborn who may become severely chilled if the temperature drops at night. Central heating or oil-filled electric radiators are probably the safest form of heating but unfortunately are not always available. Gas fires dry the air and may be dangerous if the flame blows out. Electric fires should be adequately guarded. Oil heaters should be used with care as they account for innumerable deaths from fire each year among babies and children.

Selecting Furniture

The cot is the most important piece of furniture required for a newborn baby. For the first few weeks a carry-cot is often most convenient as it can be carried everywhere and the new baby put to sleep in it during the day as well as at night. If it has a waterproof hood and cover you will be able to take the baby out in the rain. If it comes with a stand and wheels it can double as a pram. Alternatively you may like to use a basket with handles. Although lighter and easier to carry than a carry-cot, such baskets are not waterproof and therefore not very practical for outdoor use.

The baby will also feel more comfortable and secure in the first weeks of life if he is in a small cot or cradle. Moving a baby is easier if he is in a small cot, and washing small cot-sheets and blankets is less arduous than washing full-sized ones. By the time the baby is about six months old, however, a larger cot will be needed: a drop-sided wooden one is probably the most hardwearing. The side-lowering mechanism should be sturdy but move easily. The cot bars should be no more than 8 cm apart.

The cot mattress should be firm and preferably encased in a waterproof material for easy cleaning. It should fit the cot · exactly so that there is no possibility of the baby becoming wedged in a gap between mattress and cot. It should be thick enough to keep the baby warm; if the mattress you have bought is a thin one, a folded piece of blanket between the mattress and its waterproof cover will increase both the baby's warmth and his comfort. The sheets should be either flannelette or cotton. Flannelette sheets are warmer than cotton but take longer to dry. Two blankets should cover the baby: they should be light but warm; cellular blankets are now much used. Eiderdowns are optional but often used.

A pillow is unnecessary and even dangerous for a baby under one year old. There is a chance that a small baby could bury his head in a pillow and suffocate.

How much other furniture you choose to put in the baby's room will depend on personal taste, but, in the early days at least, you will probably keep the baby bath and bathing equipment in the bedroom. There are two types of baby bath in common use: one is plastic and fits into a stand, the other fits over an ordinary bath. Both of these can be used until the baby is quite big. There should also be a low chair on which you can sit to bath the baby. A trolley or table is necessary for the bathing equipment; the former can be moved easily, while the latter can be used by the toddler later on.

Cupboards are useful for clothing and for storing toys. As the child grows, a playpen may be used: this allows freedom while restricting his environment to a safe one. Some kind of baby chair will also be needed; a low chair is safer than a high one. The chair should have a firm, broad base and safety straps; its tray should be large and ideally should have rounded corners for easy cleaning.

COMFORT AND MOBILITY:
Helping the patient to move and maintain a comfortable position

COMFORT AND MOBILITY

One of your most important tasks as a volunteer is to attend to the patient's comfort. Since much of the ill person's day is spent in and around the bed, you will need to make the bed neatly and regularly — whether or not he is allowed up.

If the patient is unable to move or if his movements are restricted, it is up to you to choose the most suitable position in bed for him: you should know how to lift and move him without causing him any pain and without straining your back. Prolonged bedrest is known to be harmful: a bed-ridden patient is likely to develop pressure sores (see page 29) and there is a risk of blood clotting in his leg veins (thrombosis). Because of this risk you should turn the patient regularly and help him to take gentle exercise. The district nursing sister will guide you in all these matters.

The patient who can get up and move around should be encouraged to do so; but do not forget that even the relatively mobile patient may need help.

The Patient in Bed

Most homes have low beds. These make nursing difficult, mainly because the risk of back strain for the helper is greater. Bed blocks may be used to increase the height: these are blocks of wood placed under all four legs of the bed, but you should check frequently that they are stable.

If the patient is being nursed in a double bed it is more difficult to care for him, especially if he cannot get out of bed. If there is a single bed available, it might be worth trying to persuade him to move to it. However, if someone is sharing the bed, any nursing disadvantage will probably be outweighed by the advantage of having another person at hand during the night.

There are also adjustable beds, which can be raised or lowered by a winding handle or hydraulic foot pedal, but usually these are found only in hospitals. You lower the bed when the patient is getting in or out and raise it when bedmaking.

Bedmaking

There are many different ways of making a bed, but certain rules apply at all times:
- strip the bed neatly (see p. 28)
- mitre corners (see opposite)
- make sure that there are enough bed-clothes at the top of the bed to cover the patient when he lies down
- loosen the bedclothes over the patient's feet so that he can move his toes freely.

To make a bed, you will need:
- two sheets
- an underblanket
- two top blankets
- an eiderdown in cold weather
- as many pillows as the patient wants or his condition dictates
- two chairs back to back.

You may also be using a drawsheet (see p. 27). If you need to protect the mattress, place a piece of plastic sheeting under the drawsheet and, if necessary, another piece under the bottom sheet.

Making a cot

Making a cot is very similar to making a bed. Often it is easier: normally only one person makes a cot, stripping the bed-linen on to a chair first. It is also usually possible to lift the baby from the cot before you make it, making sure that he is comfortably wrapped in a blanket beforehand.

A pillow is unnecessary and even dangerous for a baby under one year old.

Making an empty bed

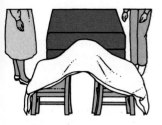

1 Make sure the bed-linen is ready folded on the chairs at the bottom of the bed in the order required. Where possible, you should work in pairs to make the bed.

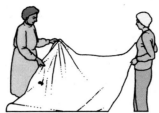

2 Cover the mattress with the underblanket. Place the bottom sheet right side up with the crease centred down the middle of the bed.

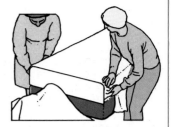

3 Tuck in the sheet along the head, then the foot of the bed. Make mitred corners (see below), pulling the sheet taut before you tuck in the sides.

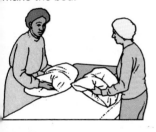

4 Put two pillows on the bed. Place the top sheet in position wrong side up, with the crease centred down the middle. Allow about a 45cm turnover and cover half the pillow.

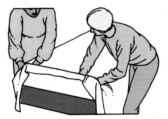

5 Tuck in the sheet at the foot of the bed. Make mitred corners and tuck in the sides. Repeat with each blanket. With the counterpane leave the sides hanging loose.

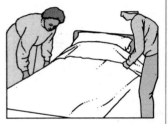

6 Loosen the bedclothes at the bottom end of the bed, and turn the excess sheet on the pillows down over the blankets and counterpane.

Making mitred corners

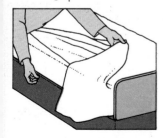

1 Pick up the edge of the sheet about 45cm from the corner of the bed.

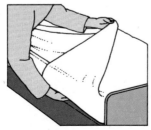

2 Tuck in the sheet hanging down between your hand and the corner.

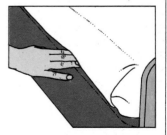

3 Allow the remaining fold of sheet to hang down and then tuck it in.

Bedmaking when the patient is in bed

It is especially important that two people make the bed together. See that the room is warm and tell the patient what you are going to do before you start. Place any clean linen on a chair near the bed. Prepare a linen bag or bucket for any soiled linen. Put two more chairs at the foot of the bed.

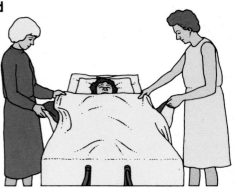

1 Loosen the bedclothes all around the mattress. Remove the counterpane by folding it in three and place it on a chair. Remove the top blanket in the same way.

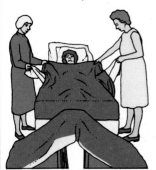

2 Slide the top sheet from under the second blanket, fold it and put it on a chair. Keep the patient well covered with the blanket and remove all but one pillow.

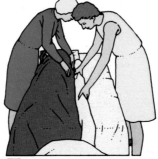

3 Roll the patient to one side of the bed. Support him while your helper brushes out any crumbs, and roll all the layers of bedlinen up to the patient's back.

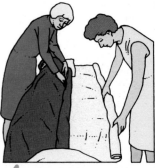

4 Straighten each layer in turn, unroll it, pull it taut and tuck it in again. Roll the patient to the other side of the bed and repeat the process.

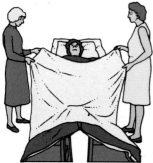

5 Tuck in all bedclothes, sit the patient forward and replace the pillows. Unfold the top sheet over the patient.

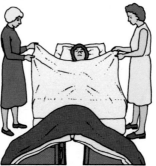

6 Remove the blanket from underneath the sheet and place it on a chair. Tuck in the sheet, allowing 45cm to turn over at the top.

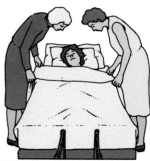

7 Replace each blanket in turn over the patient, and tuck them in. Replace the counterpane and turn down the sheet over it.

Using a Drawsheet

If the patient is in bed for more than a few days or is sweating a great deal, you may find a drawsheet useful. A rectangular piece of material about one metre wide and two metres long, a drawsheet can be made by folding a sheet in half lengthways. It is then placed on top of the bottom sheet under the patient's buttocks and allows a clean cool area to be moved under the patient without there being any need to change the bottom sheet.

   When the patient is uncomfortable and you want to adjust the drawsheet, untuck it at both ends. Pull a fresh area under the patient's buttocks and tuck in both sides again. The length of the drawsheet allows three or four fresh areas to be pulled through before the sheet needs changing.

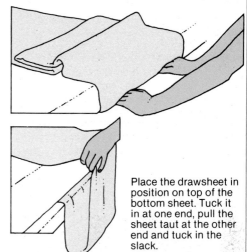

Place the drawsheet in position on top of the bottom sheet. Tuck it in at one end, pull the sheet taut at the other end and tuck in the slack.

Changing a drawsheet
Prepare a clean drawsheet by rolling it crosswise. Leave the drawsheet rolled up close to the patient's back. Tuck in the clean drawsheet and unroll it until it meets the soiled one. Roll the patient over both drawsheets before removing the soiled sheet. Tuck in the clean drawsheet.

Changing a bottom sheet
If you need to change a bottom sheet, proceed in exactly the same way. Remember to roll the clean sheet lengthwise before starting and, before tucking it in, check that its centre crease will come in the middle of the bed.

Changing a fitted sheet

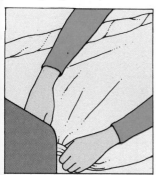

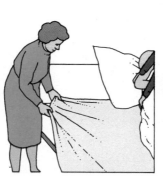

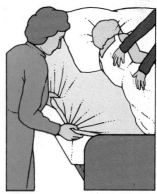

1 After putting the rolled sheet in the bed, place the top corner over the mattress, pull the sheet toward the bottom corner and ease it over.

2 Roll the patient over both the clean and the soiled sheet. Remove the soiled sheet. Pull the sheet diagonally towards the top and ease it over the corner.

3 Pull the sheet diagonally towards the bottom, bend up the mattress and ease it over the last corner. Complete bedmaking as before.

Bedmaking when the patient cannot lie flat

If the patient cannot get up for bedmaking but cannot lie flat either — probably because he is breathless — strip the bed (see below), but do not remove any pillows. Two of you should then lift the patient towards the foot of the bed. Your helper should support him while you make the top half of the bed. Remove the pillows and backrest, brush out any crumbs, remove the drawsheet and plastic sheet and place them on the chair. Roll the bottom sheet and blanket down to the patient's back, and change them or tuck them in again. Replace the plastic sheet and drawsheet and tuck them in. Support the patient while your helper tucks in the bedclothes on her side. Replace the backrest and pillows.

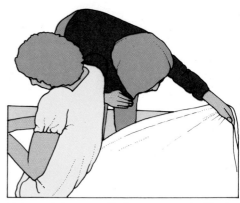

If the patient cannot lie flat, she must be lifted down the bed and supported while the sheets are changed. If you are making the bed on your own with fitted sheets, you support the patient with one arm while you invert the corner of the sheet over your other hand before easing it over the corner of the mattress.

Stripping a bed

Two people should work together to strip a bed efficiently. Fold each layer of bedlinen neatly into three before removing it from the bed. Make sure that the folded linen is placed tidily on two chairs in the order required to remake the bed.

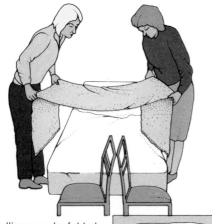

Bedlinen can be folded into three according to the preference of the people making the bed. Two common methods of folding are illustrated here.

Using a continental quilt

Continental quilts are increasing in popularity: they are warm, light, mould themselves to the body and do not slip off the bed like an eiderdown. They come filled with down, a mixture of feather and down, or man-made fibres, and have washable covers. Quilts come in various sizes: for maximum comfort use the largest.

If a continental quilt suits the patient, bedmaking is greatly simplified. However, it is important to make the bed for the patient as often as you would normally. It is tempting to think that a continental quilt merely needs to be plumped up occasionally; in fact the filling tends to collect at the bottom of the quilt, while the patient needs the pleasure of returning to a freshly made bed in the same way as any other patient.

You make the bed in the usual way. Often a fitted sheet is used, while the quilt replaces all the bedding on top of the patient. Shake the quilt so that its filling is evenly distributed and let it fall neatly on top of the pillows and bottom sheet. Avoid using a counterpane as it flattens the quilt and reduces the warmth created by the trapped air.

Pressure Areas

Whenever you sit or lie down you are compressing the skin and the underlying tissues between the bed or chair and your bones. But the compression is never so prolonged as to cause damage, because the pressure of the nerve endings in the skin causes healthy people to move frequently, even when asleep. However, if weakness, paralysis or unconsciousness makes movement impossible, the pressure may be enough to cut off the blood supply to the underlying tissues. They then die and the skin ulcerates. The ulcers are known as pressure sores. Common sites for pressure sores are: the back of the head; the shoulders; the elbows; the base of the spine; the buttocks; the sides of the hip; the knees; and the heels.

Preventing pressure sores

There are several things you can do for a patient to help prevent pressure sores. Improve the general health and the body's healing power with adequate protein and vitamin C (see page 60). Change his position regularly — about every two hours. Keep the skin over the vulnerable area clean and dry, and be careful not to damage the skin when giving a bedpan. Make sure the bottom sheet is kept dry, taut and free from crumbs. Avoid friction: do not rub the area, and always lift the patient up the bed. Relieve pressure on specific areas with pillows.

Apart from the inability to move and general debility, several other factors contribute to pressure sores:
- moisture next to the skin
- wrinkles or crumbs in the bed
- friction.

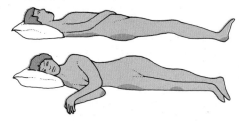

The tinted areas indicate the parts of the body most vulnerable to pressure in a patient who is sitting or lying for long periods of time.

If the patient is paralysed or incontinent, further measures can be taken. He may find that sitting on a sorbo ring or water cushion relieves pressure on the buttocks. Barrier cream may be used if he is incontinent. He may be helped by a ripple bed (alternating pressure mattress). This consists of a mattress of corrugated polythene, with an electric pump constantly inflating and deflating certain sections, so relieving pressure. Some pumps are noisy and disturb the patients; others dislike the movement. An alternative is a water bed. This is a mattress filled with water, which moves with the patient and so relieves pressure.

Treating pressure sores

If pressure sores occur, it becomes even more important to turn the patient regularly. Sores must be treated as surgical wounds. The doctor may remove dead tissue and pack the wound with gauze, which is either dry or soaked in a solution that aids healing. The pack allows the wound to heal from below upwards. The wound may also be treated with ultraviolet light or other special measures.

The patient's general health must be improved; it is essential for him to eat a balanced diet with protein and vitamin C.

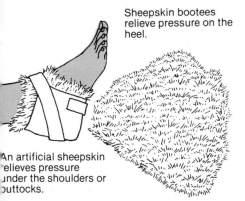

Sheepskin bootees relieve pressure on the heel.

An artificial sheepskin relieves pressure under the shoulders or buttocks.

Positions for Bedrest

There are five basic positions for bedrest, all of which can be modified to suit individual needs. The patient's condition may dictate the best position for him, but his comfort is a prime consideration.

The upright position

The patient sits up with the back supported by several pillows, or by pillows and a backrest. Two of the pillows may be used to support his arms and a footrest used to prevent him from slipping down the bed.

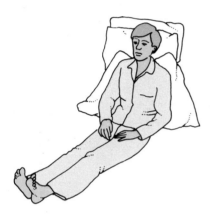

The semi-recumbent position

Three or four pillows support the patient's back. This is a comfortable position, allowing the patient to see around him and to eat and drink without strain.

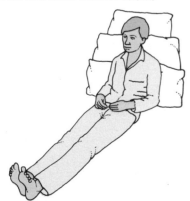

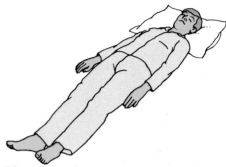

The recumbent position

The patient lies flat on his back with one or two pillows. This can be restful and allows him to turn on to his side.

The prone position

The patient lies face down with pillows to support him. This position is used for soreness of the back or buttocks.

The recovery position

This is used for the unconscious patient, who lies with his lower leg stretched out behind him, and his upper leg bent in front of him. His shoulders are tilted so that his lower arm is also behind him while his upper arm is bent in front. His head is turned to prevent the tongue blocking the airway.

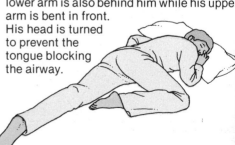

Aids to Comfort in Bed

Backrests: When the patient is sitting up his back needs to be supported, and a backrest reduces the pillows required.

Footrests: It may be necessary to support the patient's feet to prevent him from slipping down the bed. In a long illness a foot support is also used to keep the foot at right angles to the leg.

Orthopaedic boards: Patients with back problems find it difficult to lie comfortably on a soft bed. The bed can be made rigid by one long board, or a series of boards, placed across the base under the mattress.

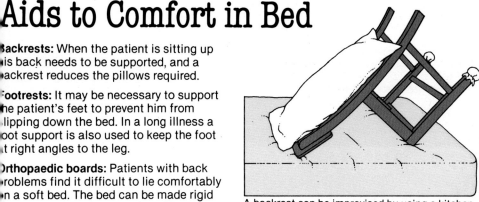

A backrest can be improvised by using a kitchen chair in conjunction with pillows. You can prevent the front legs of the chair from scratching the wall by covering them with a duster or towel.

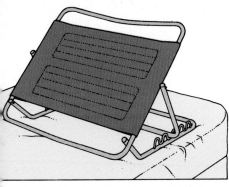

This standard backrest is widely available for use in the home.

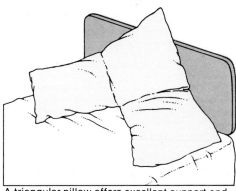

A triangular pillow offers excellent support and is much appreciated by sufferers from backache.

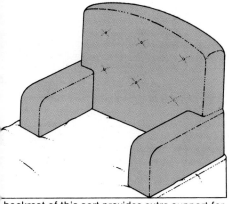

A backrest of this sort provides extra support for the arms.

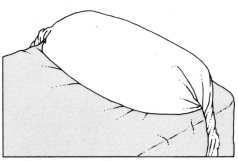

A soft footrest can either be a bolster or a pillow wrapped in a sheet.

Moving the Patient

Whenever a patient needs to be moved, you must think carefully about both his needs and your own.

The lifter: Moving a patient involves physical effort and may cause you injury if he is too heavy. You may have to arrange the care so that lifting can be done when help is available, or else make sure of some mechanical aid. There are certain points always to bear in mind when you are lifting a patient:

• clear the floor space
• keep your back straight: avoid arching it backwards or forwards

• bend your knees, not your back
• make your thigh muscles do the work
• wear supporting shoes with low heels.

The patient: Tell the patient what you are about to do so that he can cooperate. While you are moving him, always lift him up the bed; never drag him, as this will damage his skin. Make sure always to turn him towards you rather than away, as in this way you have better control.

The following pages show a selection of lifts for different conditions, all designed to protect you from injury.

Sitting the patient up

You will want to sit the patient up for meals and as a change of position, but this is also the first step in lifting him or moving him from the bed to a chair.

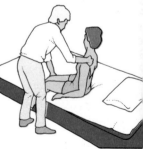

2 Keeping your arms straight, sit back on your heels. Your body weight lifts the patient to the sitting position.

1 Fold the patient's arms across her waist. Place your inside knee on the bed level with her hip and your outside foot on the floor in line with her waist. With your knee bent, put both hands under her shoulder blades.

3 With one hand supporting the patient's back, help her to swing her legs over the side of the bed. Help her to put on a dressing gown and slippers.

Lifting the patient up a low bed by yourself

In the home you may frequently be required to lift a patient up a low bed by yourself.

1 Sit the patient up (see opposite). Place your inside knee on the bed well behind her and your outside foot on the floor close to the bed. The patient should hold her right wrist with her left hand, and bend one knee. Slip your hands under her arms and grasp her forearms.

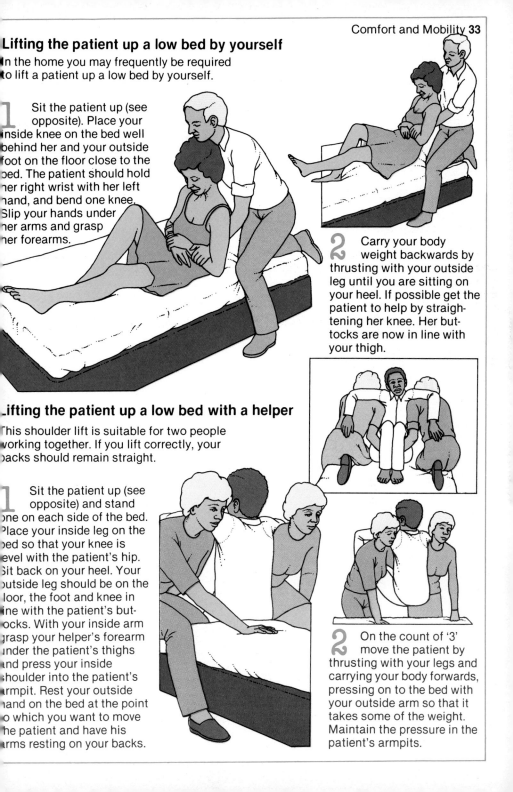

2 Carry your body weight backwards by thrusting with your outside leg until you are sitting on your heel. If possible get the patient to help by straightening her knee. Her buttocks are now in line with your thigh.

Lifting the patient up a low bed with a helper

This shoulder lift is suitable for two people working together. If you lift correctly, your backs should remain straight.

1 Sit the patient up (see opposite) and stand one on each side of the bed. Place your inside leg on the bed so that your knee is level with the patient's hip. Sit back on your heel. Your outside leg should be on the floor, the foot and knee in line with the patient's buttocks. With your inside arm grasp your helper's forearm under the patient's thighs and press your inside shoulder into the patient's armpit. Rest your outside hand on the bed at the point to which you want to move the patient and have his arms resting on your backs.

2 On the count of '3' move the patient by thrusting with your legs and carrying your body forwards, pressing on to the bed with your outside arm so that it takes some of the weight. Maintain the pressure in the patient's armpits.

Lifting the patient up a low double bed with a helper

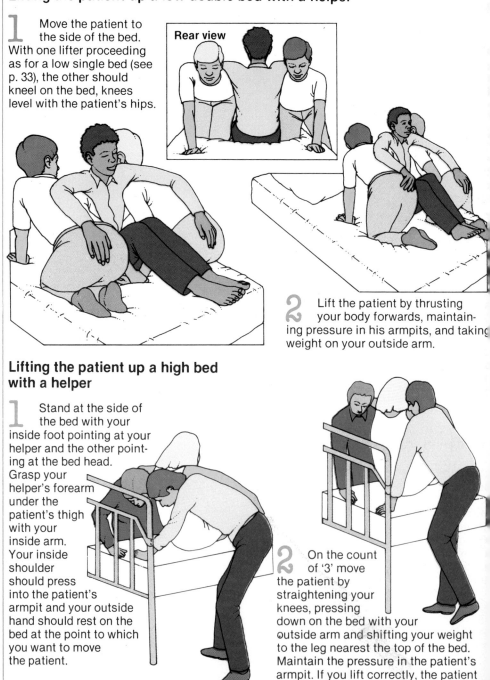

1 Move the patient to the side of the bed. With one lifter proceeding as for a low single bed (see p. 33), the other should kneel on the bed, knees level with the patient's hips.

Rear view

2 Lift the patient by thrusting your body forwards, maintaining pressure in his armpits, and taking weight on your outside arm.

Lifting the patient up a high bed with a helper

1 Stand at the side of the bed with your inside foot pointing at your helper and the other pointing at the bed head. Grasp your helper's forearm under the patient's thigh with your inside arm. Your inside shoulder should press into the patient's armpit and your outside hand should rest on the bed at the point to which you want to move the patient.

2 On the count of '3' move the patient by straightening your knees, pressing down on the bed with your outside arm and shifting your weight to the leg nearest the top of the bed. Maintain the pressure in the patient's armpit. If you lift correctly, the patient should be raised and moved backwards

Lifting the patient from bed to chair with a helper

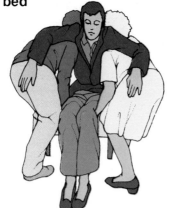

1 Place the chair in position. Sit the patient up with his legs over the side of the bed (see p. 32). Help him to put on his dressing gown and slippers. With your inside hand grasp your helper's wrist under the patient's thighs. Press your shoulders into the patient's armpits and place your outside hand flat on the bed. Your outside leg should be close to the bed with the foot pointing forwards. Your inside leg should be a little way behind with the foot pointing inwards. With your back straight and your chin tucked in, bend your hips and knees.

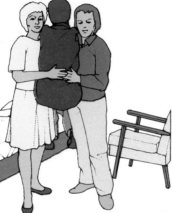

2 Lift by pressing up into the patient's armpit with your shoulder while straightening your knees and pressing firmly on the bed with your outside hand.

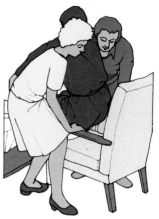

3 Support the patient's back with your outside hand as you walk towards the chair. When you reach it place your inside foot slightly in front of the chair, facing inwards, and your outside foot at the side of the chair, facing forwards. Lock your feet to prevent the chair moving. Place your outside hand on the arm of the chair. With your back straight and your knees and hips bent lower the patient gently into the chair as your elbow bends.

Helping the patient up from a chair

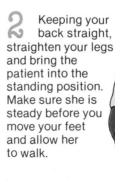

1 Stand slightly to one side of the patient and put one foot in front of hers to stop her sliding forwards. Make sure the chair cannot move. Bend your legs at the knee and place your hands under her armpits.

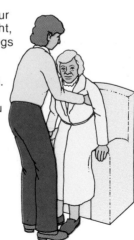

2 Keeping your back straight, straighten your legs and bring the patient into the standing position. Make sure she is steady before you move your feet and allow her to walk.

Encouraging Greater Mobility

Many patients recovering from a serious illness or an operation need help at first with walking and moving about. Elderly patients may also need help to a greater or lesser degree, as may the paralysed and handicapped. It is important to try and judge how much help the individual patient needs, and make it available to him without making him more dependent than necessary.

Helping the patient up stairs

You may need to steady the patient on the stairs by taking his arm on the side opposite the banister or wall. Make sure he is not wearing anything loose that could trail and trip him. Ideally his shoes should provide him with some support.

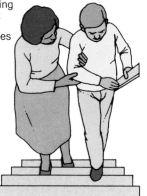

If the patient is extremely unsteady or the staircase exceptionally narrow, stand behind her and support her by putting one hand under each armpit.

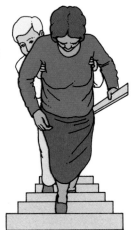

Helping the patient to walk

Patients recovering from a stroke that has temporarily paralysed one side of the body need special help.

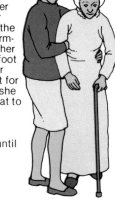

Stand at the patient's weaker side. Support her with one arm round her waist from behind and the other hand under her armpit from in front. Block her feet with your forward foot and prepare to use your knee to provide support for her weaker knee when she puts weight on it. Repeat to the patient:
● stick forward
● weak leg forward
● strong leg forward until the rhythm is well established.

Helping the patient into the car

The patient who needs to visit the doctor or hospital for treatment may need help with getting in and out of the car — especially if he is spastic, arthritic, or partially paralysed

Open the car door wide and wind down the window. Help the patient into the car while holding the door open and protecting her head from the window frame. Get the patient to grasp the car door and twist round to sit down backwards. Lift her feet in if necessary. Reverse the procedure to help the patient out.

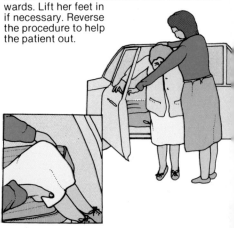

Aids to Walking

If you are not actually helping the patient as he walks with an aid, keep an eye on him. Try and see that he finishes his walk in front of the chair he wants to sit in with the back of his legs touching it. Remove the walking aid, and let him turn slightly towards his stronger side and put his stronger hand on the chair arm or his hand on the seat before sitting down.

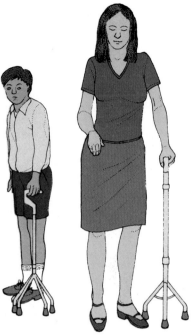

A stick with a rubber ferrule is ideal for a patient who only needs a little support or a boost to confidence.

A zimmer walking frame is ideal for someone who has to support some of his weight on his hands.

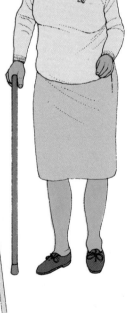

Tripods and quadrupeds are adjustable in height. They provide balanced support for those patients who need it.

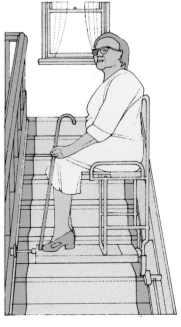

In the case of a permanent disability or condition such as breathlessness, it may be possible to install a stair lift on which the patient can stand or sit to ride up and down stairs. The social services will advise on this and in some areas will provide financial help.

The Patient in a Wheelchair

As a volunteer or helper in the home, you may find that you have to care for a patient in a wheelchair. The amount of help you will be required to give will depend on the type of patient involved. The disabled person confined permanently to a wheelchair will be very familiar with the way to use it and will probably instruct you about the specific help he needs, if any. But a temporarily incapacitated person of any age or a frail, elderly person may have to use a wheelchair for a while, yet may not be expert at handling it. This category of patient is more likely to appreciate help.

Types of wheelchair

There are many different types of wheelchair, so before handling one you should examine it carefully. Note the position of the wheels and brakes, and establish whether the armrests and footrests are fixed or movable. Two common types of wheelchair are illustrated here.

You may be involved in the care of a disabled patient who is moved from an ordinary to an electric wheelchair. Electric wheelchairs are usually operated from a lever on the armrest and run on batteries that can be recharged overnight from the mains. These chairs are expensive but offer the patient a large measure of independence. If you are helping a patient adjust to one, bear in mind that the controls are sensitive and require a degree of skill.

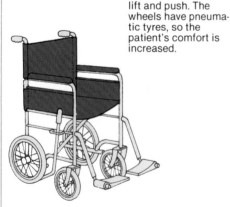

This type of chair must be pushed, but occupies less space than a self-propelling one. It is also lighter, and therefore easier to lift and push. The wheels have pneumatic tyres, so the patient's comfort is increased.

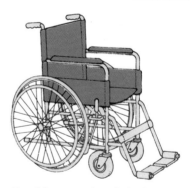

This type of chair is in common use. It has two large and two small wheels. The outer rim on the large wheels makes it possible for the patient to wheel himself.

Helping the patient into a car

When you are helping the patient from a wheelchair to a car or vice versa, make sure that the brakes of both car and chair are fully on; take note of how the patient wishes to be moved, and keep any clothing or blankets clear of the wheels. Do not hurry the patient or push the chair so fast that he is frightened of being pushed out.

Pushing a wheelchair down a kerb

It is important not to startle or jar the patient in a wheelchair when negotiating a kerb. You will be successful as long as you take care to remain in complete control. With your foot on the chair's tipping lever hold the chair firmly and tip it back. Lower it slowly and gently down the kerb, making sure both back wheels touch the ground at the same time.

WASHING AND BATHING:
Helping the patient to keep his body clean

WASHING AND BATHING

The human body is covered with skin, which is a living tissue constantly renewed, the outer layers flaking away as they die. The skin contains sweat glands, sebaceous glands, hair, blood vessels and nerves. The sweat glands help to control body temperature: as the sweat evaporates it cools the skin. The sebaceous glands lubricate the skin and keep it supple. The hairs trap air: in man this is not very important, but it provides many animals with vital warmth. The blood vessels bring nourishment to the skin and carry away waste. The nerves provide information about temperature, pressure and touch.

The feverish patient sweats profusely and quickly becomes hot, sticky, and uncomfortable. This is because the sweat glands in his skin are more active than usual during illness. A regular part of your nursing care will be to help him keep his body clean; in so doing you are removing stale sweat and allowing the glands to secrete freely. Try and assess how much

help the individual patient needs and plan your care accordingly, offering any aids that might be useful. Be prepared to wash, shave and bath the patient, and help care for his mouth, nails, hair and eyes if this proves necessary.

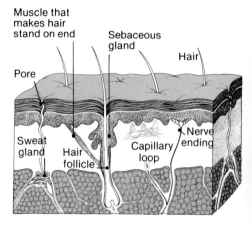

Muscle that makes hair stand on end
Sebaceous gland
Hair
Pore
Sweat gland
Hair follicle
Capillary loop
Nerve ending

Bathing

If the patient is mobile enough, he can bath in the bathroom, perhaps with the help of bathing aids. If the patient is confined to bed or very inactive, he can be bathed in bed. A daily bath is ideal — though it is as well to check how often the patient would normally bath. Many patients, especially the elderly, are nervous of bathing. In these circumstances a good wash down can be just as adequate.

Bathing provides you with the opportunity to observe the patient carefully; if you notice any changes in the colour and appearance of the skin, you should report them immediately.

Bathing in the bathroom
Make sure that the bathroom is warm and that any windows are closed. Gather together soap, flannels, towels, talcum powder and any clean clothes that may be

wanted. Run cold water first, then add the hot and mix thoroughly. Now tell the patient that his bath is ready and, if necessary, help him to the bathroom. You may need to offer him help with getting in and out of the bath (see p. 42). Patients who need a lot of help should use a bath seat (opposite).

Some patients may need help with washing and drying, while others may be well enough to be left alone. A patient left on his own, however, should not lock the door, and should have a bell within reach. Never leave a child alone in the bathroom.

After the patient has left the bathroom, clean the bath, hang up the flannels and towels to dry and leave the room tidy.

A person confined to bed can still be washed all over. This is known as a bed or blanket bath and includes caring for the nails, eyes, hair, mouth and teeth (see pages 43-47).

Aids to Bathing

A handrail or a bath seat may make it possible for a frail or elderly person to bath alone. If you are caring for a heavy or disabled patient, you might borrow a hoist. This is a device used to lift people into the bath. The correct type must be recommended by a competent therapist, who will also teach you how to operate it.

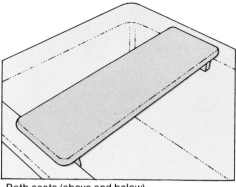

Bath seats (above and below) help patients who find it hard to get down to the bottom of the bath.

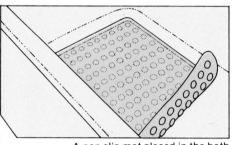

A non-slip mat placed in the bath is held firm by suction pads.

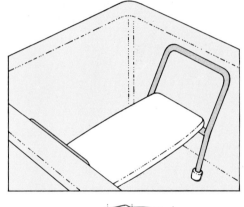

There are many different sorts of handrail (examples left and below). Some can be dangerous and the most expensive are not necessarily the best. Get expert advice before choosing one.

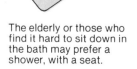

The elderly or those who find it hard to sit down in the bath may prefer a shower, with a seat.

Getting in and out of the Bath

The two methods of helping the patient into the bath illustrated here are alternatives. Which you choose will largely depend on the position of the bath and the facilities available to you.

To help a patient out of the bath, follow the procedures illustrated below in reverse. If the patient finds it hard to get up, drain the water, cover him with a warm towel and step into the bath yourself. Bend your knees, place your hands under his armpits, straighten your legs and lift him upright.

Method one

1 Stand behind the patient and get him to grasp his wrist with his other hand. Slip your hands under his armpits and grasp his forearms in front of his waist.

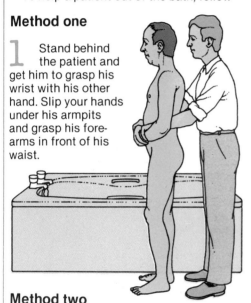

2 Let the patient step into the bath. Keeping your back straight, bend your knees and lower him on to a bath seat or the floor of the bath.

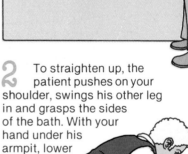

Method two

1 Stand facing the patient sideways on to the bath and place your hand under his arm. Help him lift his inner leg into the bath.

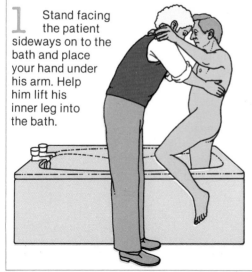

2 To straighten up, the patient pushes on your shoulder, swings his other leg in and grasps the sides of the bath. With your hand under his armpit, lower him gradually into the bath.

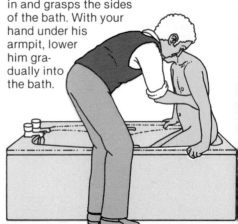

Giving a Bed Bath

Make sure that the bedroom is warm and the windows closed. You will need:

- a bowl of hot water
- soap
- two towels
- a face flannel
- a body flannel
- talcum powder
- a deodorant
- a change of clothing
- a brush and comb.

Remove the top bedclothes, leaving the patient covered with a blanket. Help to take off pyjamas or nightdress and place a towel underneath each part as you wash it to protect the bed. First wash, rinse and dry the face, neck and ears; if the patient is well enough he may do this for himself.

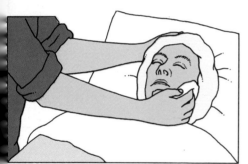

Ask the patient if she likes soap on her face. Using a face flannel and towel, wash, rinse, and dry the face, neck and ears.

Wash, rinse, and dry one arm from the armpit to the fingers, then repeat with the other. Let the patient rinse his hands in the bowl of water. Wash and dry the patient's chest and abdomen. Powder under his arms or use a deodorant if appropriate. Wash and dry each leg in turn: when possible flex his knee and rinse each foot in the bowl after washing: this is very refreshing. Many patients can wash the groin and genital area for themselves, if you hold the blanket out of their way. Very ill or unconscious patients will not be able to do this, so you must do it for them. You may find it

easier to wash this area when the patient is lying on his side. You roll him on to his side to wash his back.

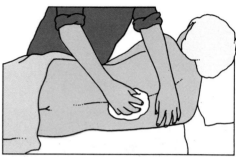

Roll the patient on to her side so that her back can be washed. If you are alone the patient should turn towards you to minimize the risk of her falling out of bed.

As you wash the patient, keep him covered as much as possible. Change the water whenever it cools and after the genital area has been washed. Use talcum powder and toilet water if the patient likes them. When you have finished, help the patient to put on clean nightwear. (If possible keep separate clothing for night-time.)

After bathing the patient, help him to clean his teeth, brush his hair, and to shave if necessary (see p. 44). You may need to help the female patient with her make-up. Remake the bed, before clearing the room and opening a window.

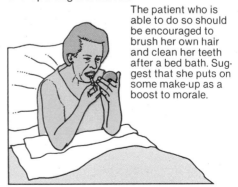

The patient who is able to do so should be encouraged to brush her own hair and clean her teeth after a bed bath. Suggest that she puts on some make-up as a boost to morale.

Shaving

A man who shaves regularly will find it both uncomfortable and embarrassing when stubble grows. If he is unable to shave himself, then you must do it for him.

Before you start, assess the patient's condition and judge how much help he needs. Ask him what kind of razor he normally uses — switching from an electric to a safety razor will cause him discomfort for several days. Also find out in which direction he shaves: the bristles grow according to the direction of shaving, so going against the normal lay causes pulling and tenderness.

Plan your care according to how much the patient can do for himself. Protect him and the bed with towels. Wash and dry his face in the usual way.

Using a safety razor

Lather the chin, rubbing the soap well in: this softens the beard and makes the shave more comfortable. If the patient cannot manage to do it for himself, re-lather and shave him in the direction he has indicated. Take long, firm strokes and rinse the razor frequently. When you have finished, rinse the patient's face and dry it thoroughly. Use after-shave lotion if he would like it. Clear everything away and clean the razor.

Using an electric razor

If the patient uses an electric razor, check that it is clean. Shave the patient's face in the correct direction before you wash it. Allow the razor to cut the stubble, never scrub across the face. Pre-electric or after-shave lotions may be used if the patient likes them. Finally, clear everything away and clean the razor.

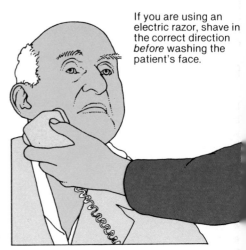

If you are using an electric razor, shave in the correct direction *before* washing the patient's face.

When using a safety razor, shave in long, firm strokes in the direction preferred by the patient, rinsing the razor frequently in between strokes.

Washing

Bear in mind that, as well as bathing, the patient needs to wash at other times. Washing his hands and face often refreshes an ill person and makes him feel more comfortable. (He should also wash his hands after using a bedpan or commode, or going to the lavatory.)

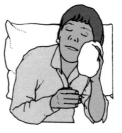

Make a point of offering the patient confined to bed a face flannel and a bowl of warm water several times a day.

Caring for the Nails

You will have the opportunity to notice if the patient's nails need attention while you are bathing him. You may find you have to use a nail brush to keep his nails clean, and you should also remember to cut the nails regularly: fingernails should be cut or filed to the shape of the finger, while toenails should be cut straight across. The female patient may enjoy a manicure if you have time — and nail varnish is often a boost to morale.

It is not uncommon for elderly people to have very hard and horny nails. The help of a chiropodist is invaluable in these cases: in some instances the elderly person has been housebound because of the state of his toenails and the chiropodist can, quite literally, put him on his feet again. But although health authorities are obliged to provide a chiropody service, it is often inadequate, even for the elderly. Additional foot care may be provided by a voluntary organization.

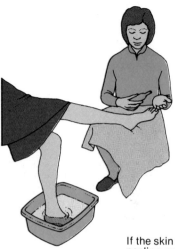

If the skin is dry and peeling, soaking the patient's feet before rubbing in a little olive or vegetable oil will help to correct this.

Caring for the Eyes

In normal health the eyes are kept moist and clean by an imperceptible film of fluid, which flows across the eyeball and drains into the nose. In illness, however, the eyes may become dry, sore and occasionally even infected. If this happens you must bathe the eyes to keep them clean.
You will need:
● a tray
● cotton wool swabs
● a bowl of clean water or a saline solution (one 5 ml spoonful of salt to 600 ml of previously boiled water)
● a paper towel or square of kitchen roll
● a paper bag for used swabs
● eye drops if prescribed (see page 74).

Help the patient into a comfortable position and tell him what you are going to do. If he can lie flat you can stand behind his head, the ideal position from which to treat the eyes. If this is not possible see that the patient's head is back and his shoulders supported. Wash your hands. Arrange the towel under his face. Dip a swab into the water or saline solution, squeeze it gently, and swab the eye from the nose outwards. Discard the swab. Repeat the procedure until both eyes are clean. Dry the surrounding skin with clean, dry swabs. Use each swab *once only* — this is vital in order to prevent cross-infection.

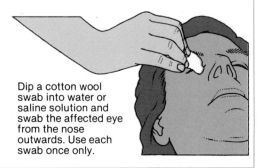

Dip a cotton wool swab into water or saline solution and swab the affected eye from the nose outwards. Use each swab once only.

Caring for the Mouth

After each meal, minute particles of food are left behind in the mouth. These particles begin to decompose and harmful bacteria flourish and multiply. As well as leaving an unpleasant taste and feeling in the mouth, these bacteria can cause tooth decay or mouth infections.

It is therefore essential to keep the mouth clean. The healthy person will clean his teeth regularly. But patients confined to bed are unable to care for their mouths without assistance. In many cases, all you need to do is to provide them with the means to clean their teeth at regular intervals. As well as toothbrush and toothpaste, give the patient a glass of water and a bowl

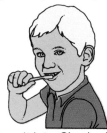

As soon as a child is old enough, get him into the habit of cleaning his teeth twice a day. Also try and restrict his intake of sticky, sweet foods.

to spit into. Check whether he prefers warm or cold water. Unless the doctor forbids it, leave a jug of water within the patient's reach and encourage him to drink.

Mouthwashes are also refreshing: offer sharp-tasting fruit juices sometimes as an alternative to brand-named varieties. In addition to cleansing, the sharp flavour of the juices encourages the glands to produce saliva, which is antiseptic and cleans the mouth. Chewing gum and small pieces of fruit — such as fresh pineapple — also cause saliva to flow.

In some cases the patient may be too ill or weak to attend to his own mouth and you must do it for him. All ill patients should have their mouths cleaned several times a day, both before and after meals. Done frequently, cleaning the mouth is simple to do and takes only a short time, but if the mouth is neglected, cleaning it becomes a difficult task for you and an ordeal for the patient.

You will need:
- a tray
- a small container holding bicarbonate of soda solution (one 5 ml spoonful of powder to 600 ml of water)
- a small container of mouthwash or water
- some orange sticks dressed with cotton wool at the ends.
- a paper towel or square of kitchen roll
- a paper bag for used swabs and sticks
- cream, lip salve or vaseline for dry lips.

Help the patient into a comfortable position and tell him what you are going to do. Wash your hands, before tucking the towel under the patient's chin. Dip the dressed stick in the solution of bicarbonate of soda and clean all the surfaces of the mouth. Discard each dressed stick as soon as it is soiled. When you have finished, swab the mouth again in the same way with mouthwash or water, to remove the somewhat unpleasant taste of bicarbonate of soda.

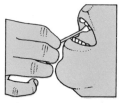

Clean the mouth from the top downwards: the gums, the teeth, the inside of the cheeks and the tongue. Clean the tongue last as pressure on it may make the patient retch.

Denture care

Get the patient to remove his dentures and place them in a container. Take them to the bathroom and brush them under cold running water. If the dentures are stained, brush them with a special denture cream or powder or soak them in a special solution. Rinse thoroughly before returning them to the patient.

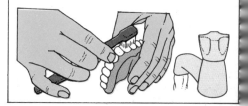

Caring for the Hair

Brush and comb the patient's hair at least twice a day, and arrange it in a simple style that is easy to manage and pleases the patient. The female patient may appreciate a pretty ribbon to match her nightdress.

Anyone who has been ill for a long period will probably need his hair washed, although dry shampooing may be sufficient. A local hairdresser may be willing to visit the home, but will usually require the patient to sit at a handbasin.

Washing hair in bed is largely a matter of helping the patient into a suitable position, covering both patient and bed with a liberal supply of waterproof material and protecting the floor with plastic sheet or newspaper. You should find out what shampoo and conditioner the patient prefers. Wash the hair thoroughly and rinse it well in clean water. Use a hair dryer if there is one available, otherwise rub the hair dry with warm towels. Finish by brushing and combing it so that it looks attractive.

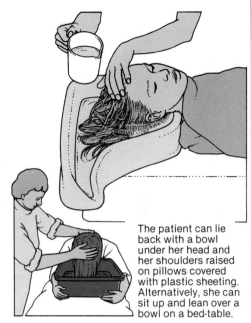

The patient can lie back with a bowl under her head and her shoulders raised on pillows covered with plastic sheeting. Alternatively, she can sit up and lean over a bowl on a bed-table.

Examining an infested head

Where living conditions are poor or the facilities for personal hygiene inadequate, hair may become infested with lice. Lice multiply quickly by laying eggs. The eggs are called nits and stick to strands of hair.

Lice can spread from one person to another, especially in crowded conditions. If an infested head is found, ask the other members of the family for permission to examine their heads. Once you have treated the condition, examine the hair regularly to check that there is no recurrence.

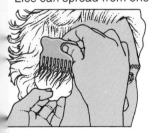

1 Having protected the patient's shoulders, dip a fine tooth-comb into disinfectant solution. With a swab in one hand, comb the hair downwards from the roots to the tip.

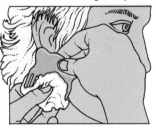

2 Wipe the comb on the swab after each stroke. Examine it carefully for lice and inspect the hair for nits. Scurf will brush out but nits stick firmly to the strands of hair.

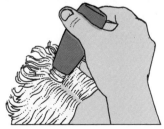

3 If lice are found, apply a chemical compound such as malathion or carbaryl. Follow the maker's instructions carefully, taking care to protect the patient's eyes from the chemicals.

Bathing the New Baby

Make sure the room is warm and close the windows. Prepare everything on a trolley or table near the bath.
You will need:

- baby cream, baby powder, baby soap
- a jar with swabs
- a change of clothing
- safety pins
- a large towel
- a bucket for soiled clothes
- a paper bag.

Fill the bath, putting the cold water in first, then adding hot until the water feels pleasantly warm to your elbow. Wash your hands and undress the baby apart from his napkin.

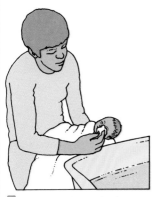

1 Wrap the baby in a towel. Wash his face with a swab or soft flannel and dry it carefully.

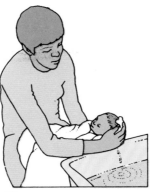

2 Lie the baby with his head towards the bath. Support his neck with one hand and rinse his hair with the other. You will not need to use soap daily.

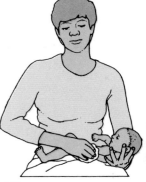

3 Pat the baby's head dry with a towel. Remove the napkin, cleaning the buttocks with swabs if it is soiled. Lather your hands and soap the baby.

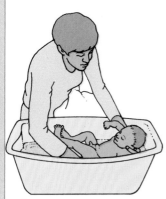

4 Lift the baby into the bath, supporting his head and shoulders with one hand and his buttocks and thighs with the other.

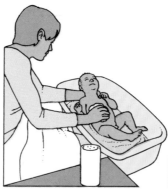

5 Still supporting the baby with the hand behind his head, rinse the soap off him with your other hand.

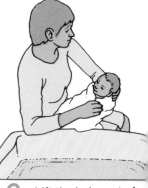

6 Lift the baby out of the bath in the same grip and wrap him in the towel. Pat him dry all over before dressing him again.

CLOTHING:
Helping the patient to dress and undress and to select clothing

CLOTHING

Choice of clothing is a very personal thing and patients and their relatives will probably have very fixed ideas about what they like and dislike. However, if illness or disability make it necessary to adapt clothing for a specific need, most people appreciate help.

This means that, as well as being able to help dress and undress the patient and offering dressing aids to make it easier for him to dress and undress himself, you should also know what special clothing is available for his particular disability. Remember that, in helping the patient select the right clothing for his condition, tact is just as important as the choice itself. Be careful not to cause embarrassment by suggesting items which are out of the patient's price range.

Dressing and Undressing

It is wise to encourage the patient to do as much for himself as he can. This may be a lengthy process if he is blind, has lost a limb or is paralysed as the result of an injury or stroke. Dressing and undressing are an important part of the patient's day: every achievement is a step towards independence. Allow the patient plenty of time for dressing and undressing and encourage him to rest at intervals.

Sleeves over arms

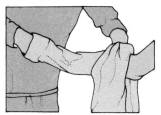

1 If one arm is injured or paralysed, deal with it first. Slip your hand through the sleeve of the garment and grasp the patient's hand.

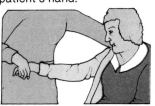

2 Gently slide the sleeve of the garment along the patient's arm.

Trousers over legs

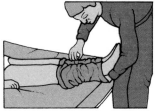

1 With the patient lying on the bed, slip the trouser legs over and along first one leg and then the other leg.

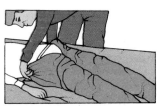

2 Pull the trousers up as far as possible and help the patient to lift his buttocks off the bed. Ease the trousers up to the waist and fasten them.

Garment over head

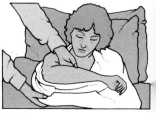

If the patient's arms both function, slip the garment first over the head then over the arms.

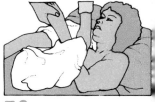

If the patient is lying down, slip her arms into the garment first, then ease the neck opening over her head. The garment needs to be fairly loose.

Aids to Dressing

Tasks that most people take for granted become impossible to carry out when a person is weak or arthritic. With the help of a few simple aids, an elderly person may find it possible to continue dressing himself and so retain his dignity.

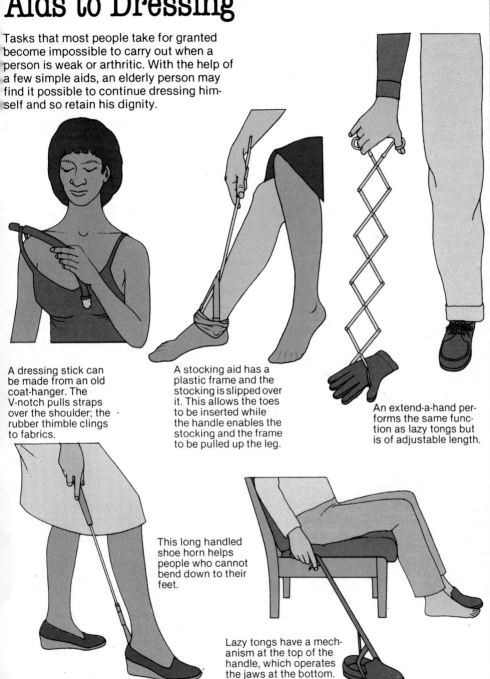

A dressing stick can be made from an old coat-hanger. The V-notch pulls straps over the shoulder; the rubber thimble clings to fabrics.

A stocking aid has a plastic frame and the stocking is slipped over it. This allows the toes to be inserted while the handle enables the stocking and the frame to be pulled up the leg.

An extend-a-hand performs the same function as lazy tongs but is of adjustable length.

This long handled shoe horn helps people who cannot bend down to their feet.

Lazy tongs have a mechanism at the top of the handle, which operates the jaws at the bottom.

Selecting Clothing

Before selecting clothing, consider any specific problems the patient may have. People who are incontinent, handicapped, confined to a wheelchair, partially sighted or who have arthritic hands, all need careful individual consideration. With a little ingenuity, many ordinary items of clothing can be adapted to individual needs.

Once you have taken the particular circumstances into account, the style of clothing selected will also depend on the weather and the kind of activity the patient is likely to undertake. Clothes should preferably all be light, easily washed and dried and require little or no ironing. Flame-resistant materials are best wherever possible, especially for the nightwear of children and incapacitated people. If the material is man-made, it should be 100 per cent polyester, which tends to melt in contact with fire; never acrylic, which will flare up.

The type and style of clothing chosen will depend very much on specific needs but it must look attractive and fit well to boost morale. Shoes should be comfortable and give support. Slippers should be discouraged, especially after a stroke. The slip-on shoe is the easiest to manage but you can buy elastic laces if the patient prefers lace-up shoes.

If the patient's clothing needs protecting at meal-times, a plastic apron or a small make-up cape may do the job unobtrusively. For the patient paralysed on one side, a dress with a protective front may be useful — the front can be added at meal-times and removed when not required.

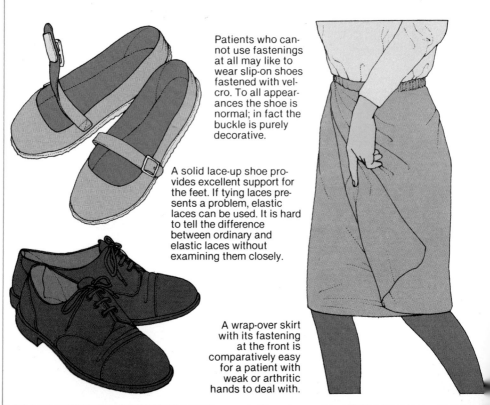

Patients who cannot use fastenings at all may like to wear slip-on shoes fastened with velcro. To all appearances the shoe is normal; in fact the buckle is purely decorative.

A solid lace-up shoe provides excellent support for the feet. If tying laces presents a problem, elastic laces can be used. It is hard to tell the difference between ordinary and elastic laces without examining them closely.

A wrap-over skirt with its fastening at the front is comparatively easy for a patient with weak or arthritic hands to deal with.

If the patient's hands are weak or rheumatic, front fastenings and wrap-over skirts are easier to deal with. Conventional fastenings can be replaced with velcro. Special braces can make it easier to take trousers on and off. These braces are attached to the middle of the back of the trousers and worn round the neck like a school satchel. To put his trousers on, the patient holds the trouser band and neck piece of the braces in one hand and steps through the braces into the trouser legs. He should then sit down to pull up his trousers as far as he can and to lift the braces over his head. When he stands up, the braces will pull the trousers up over his buttocks, with the help of his stronger hand.

Brassieres with front fastenings may help the arthritic or paralysed patient; some patients may prefer to fasten a back fastening in front and rotate it to the back. After the removal of a breast (mastectomy) a "criss cross" bra or pattern supplied by the National Health Service is the most suitable.

Women with arthritic hands may find tights easier to cope with than suspenders. Tights do exclude the air and some people find them uncomfortable. They also seem to increase the likelihood of vaginal infections but this problem can be overcome by buying single-leg tights, tights with cotton gussets or tights with no gusset, all of which allow air to circulate more freely. Garters are not a good idea, as they impede circulation. If the patient finds pulling pants up and down difficult, there is a special crotch vent knicker which she may find useful.

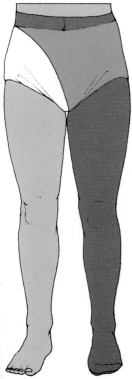

The advantages of both tights and stockings are combined in single-leg tights. These eliminate the need for suspenders, while at the same time they allow more air to circulate than ordinary tights. Like stockings, however, they only need to be replaced one at a time.

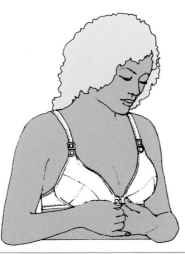

This shirt and tie look perfectly ordinary and can be bought from a department store. In fact the tie is ready-tied and fastened to the shirt collar with velcro.

Like the wrap-over skirt, a front-fastening brassiere simplifies an ordinary daily task that can seem extremely difficult to the patient with weak or arthritic hands.

Clothing for the incontinent

Incontinence brings many problems, but garments that open easily, have wrap-over backs or conceal drainage bags alleviate some of them. For those female patients whose problem is the inability to wait rather than true incontinence, French knickers may prove easier to manage than many other underclothes.

Garments with wrap-over backs have two flaps that can be moved from under the buttocks when the patient is sitting or lying, so avoiding soiling. Nightdresses, dressing gowns and dresses are available with wrap-over backs, in a number of pleasant and easily-washed materials. These clothes give comfort and security to the incontinent, and are labour-saving for those providing care.

For men, velcro fastenings and elastic waist-bands make trousers easier to cope with. Special braces (see page 53) mean that trousers can be dropped and pulled up with one hand. Suits can be adapted for easy movement and flies enlarged to cope with urinals and other appliances. For the incontinent man, a long open-back shirt is available; for those wearing pyjamas for long periods the U-shaped crotch and raglan sleeve make movement easier.

Many normal garments can be adapted: long zips or velcro fastenings can be added; dresses can open right down the front; a skirt may be opened down both sides and the front panel secured around the waist with tapes, allowing the back panel to be pulled down easily. Some WRVS centres and other organizations may give help with alterations. The district nursing sister, social worker for the disabled or Citizens Advice Bureau will be able to provide you with information about where special clothing may be bought.

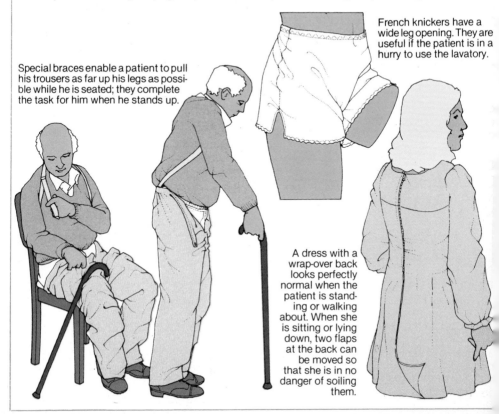

French knickers have a wide leg opening. They are useful if the patient is in a hurry to use the lavatory.

Special braces enable a patient to pull his trousers as far up his legs as possible while he is seated; they complete the task for him when he stands up.

A dress with a wrap-over back looks perfectly normal when the patient is standing or walking about. When she is sitting or lying down, two flaps at the back can be moved so that she is in no danger of soiling them.

Dressing the New Baby

In the first months of life babies do not like to be naked. Without wrapping of some sort they feel insecure. Their intense dislike of being undressed can make dressing and undressing an ordeal for both you and the baby. Because of this you should proceed with as little fuss as possible, remembering to pull the clothes rather than the baby's limbs wherever possible. If the baby seems very unhappy when he is naked, however securely you are holding him, try leaving a clean folded napkin on his tummy while you are removing the rest of his clothes. The contact may be enough to keep him calm.

It is a good idea to change the bottom half of the baby's clothing with the baby lying flat on a hard surface, as this way he is supported and both your hands are free. The top half usually causes more problems: for this proceeding with the baby on your lap is probably best.

Undressing the baby

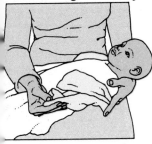 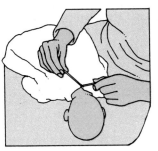 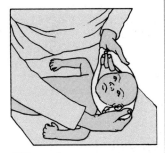

1 Supporting the baby's head with one arm, ease first one sleeve of his cardigan, then the other, over his arm.

2 Turn him on to his front, face down on your lap, while you undo any strings or buttons on his gown before removing it.

3 Turn him round again. After sliding his arms out of his vest, stretch the neck opening and pull his vest over his head.

Dressing the baby

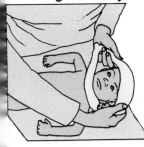 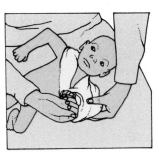 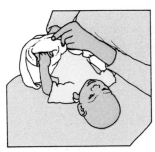

1 Stretch the opening of the baby's vest as much as possible before putting it over his head, so that he does not feel he is being smothered.

2 Put your hand through each rolled-up sleeve and guide his hand through first one sleeve and then the other.

3 Repeat the process for his gown or for any other garment that has to go over the baby's arms.

Selecting Children's Clothing

The new baby

New babies are usually given far too much clothing, most of which they rapidly outgrow. The basic rule to follow is to keep clothing simple: on the whole you should avoid fussy garments and make use of flame-resistant garments where possible.

Vests should be well-made and non-shrink. The envelope neck is the most appropriate type for small babies, as it slips over the neck easily. One-piece garments are practical and warm, but do not misunderstand the term "stretch suit". This type of garment is intended to stretch only within the age range for which it is specified and will not grow with the baby indefinitely.

Raglan sleeves make dressing and undressing easier. Lacy garments are best avoided as there is a danger of small fingers becoming trapped in holes. Drawstrings should be avoided for the same reason. Buttons should be securely fixed as loose ones can be swallowed or pushed into the nose or ears. If a baby is kicking vigorously, especially at night, with the result that he is cold and uncovered, a sleeping-bag outfit is very practical. Warm outdoor clothing in winter is essential, especially for the head, from which a baby can lose a lot of heat fast.

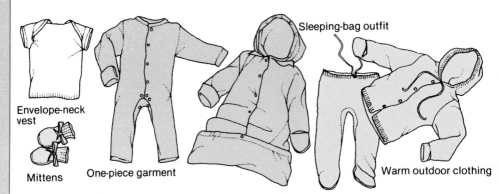

Envelope-neck vest

Mittens

One-piece garment

Sleeping-bag outfit

Warm outdoor clothing

The older child

It is outside the scope of this book to discuss clothing for healthy children in detail. Certain general principles should be mentioned, however: clothing should be roomy, with wide armholes and plenty of legroom, lightweight while suitable for the time of year. Tight bands and belts are best avoided: garments that fasten in the front make it easier for a child to learn how to dress and undress himself. Buying new clothes one size too big is a false economy: when the clothes are new they do not fit properly, and by the time they fit they need replacing. Stretch materials are practical, comfortable and come in a wide range of colours.

Shoes

A young child does not need shoes until he is walking out of doors. Before this going barefoot will give him a better sense of grip.

Shoes for everyday wear should preferably be made of leather and be at least 1½ cm longer than the child's foot. The front end of the shoes should be rounded not pointed. Lace-ups are best as they give most support, though well-made sandals are light and cool in warm weather. Since shoes should be both long enough and wide enough for the foot, proper fitting and regular checking are essential.

EATING AND DRINKING:
Helping the patient to take an adequate diet and feed himself

EATING AND DRINKING

Food and drink are necessary to life and health. They also give a great deal of pleasure. Everyone enjoys good food, attractively served in pleasant surroundings. Even the ill person whose appetite is not great will often respond to the right sorts of food served to him in the right quantity at the right time.

If you are concerned with preparing and serving food to a patient, it will help you to understand the basic principles of good nutrition. You should know how the body makes use of food, what basic nutrients are needed in a balanced diet, and in what foods they are found. This knowledge will help you to prepare balanced meals according to the needs of the patient. If you also take care to present meals attractively so that they look appetising, you have a good chance of overcoming any reluctance of the patient to eat caused by the loss of his appetite.

The Importance of a Balanced Diet

To eat well means to eat a variety of foods containing the different nutrients, which are the basic substances found in food. The nutrients in food are used by the body:
- to provide energy for movement
- to provide heat so that the body temperature remains stable between 36°C and 37°C
- to provide for normal growth
- to replace cells as they wear out or are destroyed by illness.

The principles of good nutrition are based on knowing a person's needs and on satisfying them with foods containing these essentials. You must take into consideration the person's age, sex and occupation. Children and young people need more protein for growth; men need more food than women; the young and active at work and play use more energy and more food than those who lead a quieter life; the manual worker uses more energy and more food than the typist. Climate is also a factor: in cold weather, people need more food to keep warm.

Bearing in mind these principles, you can work out the right quantity of food for a particular person. The new unit of measurement is the joule, which has now replaced the calorie: 4.18 joules = 1 calorie. A person's needs are calculated at so many joules a day. All foods have a known joule value and the overall number of joules required should be distributed between the different nutrient categories: proteins, fats and carbohydrates. Although the bulk of a person's daily intake comes from carbohydrates, it is vital that adequate amounts of protein are taken every day. (See the chart on pages 60-61 for more information about these nutrient categories.) With the addition of fluids and enough fresh food to supply the vitamins and minerals, the diet is balanced.

Some people eat an unbalanced diet through ignorance; others do so through lack of time, money, imagination, or self-indulgence. Low-income groups, such as the elderly, cannot afford expensive protein foods like meat or fish or the added cost of cooking them. They resort to the cheaper carbohydrate foods, which are easily prepared or bought ready to eat. The working girl or busy housewife may also use pre-packaged convenience foods to save time but many of these foods are high in carbohydrate at the expense of protein. Such foods fill the stomach without providing adequate nourishment for the body.

Dieticians calculate food requirements in a careful and scientific manner and, in some illnesses, diet must be strictly regulated. For practical everyday eating, exact calculations of food requirements are unnecessary. The only thing that matters is that the diet should be varied and interesting.

Nutrition in Illness

For a number of conditions the doctor will order a specific diet, which must, of course, be followed carefully. In many other cases, the doctor will simply indicate the type of diet to give the patient. You then have freedom of choice within the prescribed limits.

Types of Diet

Fluid diets

The patient is only given fluids. An adult should have at least 3 litres (about 5 pints) a day and at least half of this should be milk. Milk is a unique fluid because it contains every food requirement, with the exception of vitamin C and iron. Some patients will drink milk as it is, others prefer a flavouring, such as Ovaltine, Horlicks, Bovril, cocoa, coffee or chocolate. If the patient is very thin or undernourished or if he is likely to be taking fluids only for some time, one of the protein preparations such as Complan can be added to the milk.

To complement the milk the patient may have water, fruit juice, thin soup or any other suitable drink such as Bovril. It may be helpful to remember that since an average cup holds about 150ml of fluid, 20 cups will be needed to give the required daily intake of 3 litres (3000ml).

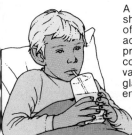

A child on a fluid diet should be given plenty of milk flavoured according to his preference. Brightly coloured straws and a variety of different glasses and cups will encourage him to drink as much as he needs to.

Light diets

A light diet consists of easily digestible foods such as fish, white meat, eggs, milk, bread and butter. Vegetables and fruit or fruit juice are given in small quantities but fried foods should be avoided. A light diet can seem boring but a little ingenuity works wonders and attractive presentation of the food may solve the problem.

Special diets

Many special diets play an important part in the treatment of a disease, such as diabetes. In this disease, the body is unable to store any reserves of glucose. Carbohydrates are therefore given in limited quantities, just adequate for the body's immediate needs. If the diet is not followed, the patient may lose consciousness; if he is not then treated he may die. If you are caring for a diabetic patient, you will usually be supplied with a diet sheet but, if there is any difficulty, you should seek the advice of the doctor, district nursing sister or health visitor.

Another common special diet is the low-joule diet, prescribed for the patient who is overweight. A large number of people get into the habit of eating too much. There is evidence that unhealthy eating habits are learned in infancy: over the years there can be a steady increase in weight. Overweight people are much more likely to develop illnesses of various kinds, such as joint and back pain, coronary artery disease and high blood pressure. Prevention is always better than cure, so that anyone who has a tendency to be overweight would be wise to restrict his total carbohydrate intake and be careful not to eat between meals. Once a diet is prescribed for someone who is seriously overweight, however, carbohydrate foods are drastically reduced. A diet sheet is prepared for the patient containing approximately 4000 joules a day. Bread, potatoes and sugar are severely restricted and replaced by salads and fresh fruit. The main purpose is to re-educate the eating habits, as most overweight people positively enjoy the carbohydrate element in their food and do not like to be restricted to items which they probably regard as inadequately 'filling'.

CATEGORIES OF NUTRIENT

Nutrient	In which foods	Importance to body
Proteins 8-10% of total daily joule requirement	Meat, fish, eggs, milk, cheese, peas, beans, nuts, cereals.	Proteins are necessary throughout life for the replacement of worn-out cells. They also promote growth, so they are essential for pregnant women and children. During a long illness or after a serious operation the body is severely deprived of protein. The body cannot store protein, so some must be eaten daily.
Carbohydrates 65-80% of total daily joule requirement	Sugar and all products sweetened with it (such as sweets, cakes, puddings, and jam); potatoes and some other root vegetables; bread, flour, cereals.	All starches and sugars are broken down into glucose by the body to provide heat and energy. They are essential in moderation, but any excess is turned into fat by the body.
Fats 5-10% of total daily joule requirement	Butter, margarine, cooking fat, cooking oil, lard, dripping, meat fat, cream, milk, cheese, egg yolk, olive oil, fish oils, salad cream.	Fats are a concentrated source of warmth and energy. People tend to eat fatty foods more in the winter, but it is easy to take them in excess at any time: a summer meal of cheese salad with lashings of salad cream contains a large amount of fat.
Vitamins Vitamins are essential for good health and are present in many foods in minute quantities. Lack of them leads to deficiency diseases. Anyone eating a well-balanced diet will automatically take in enough vitamins. If the patient's diet is inadequate, the doctor will prescribe a vitamin supplement. It is important to make sure the patient does not forget to take the supplement.		
Vitamin A	Liver and fish liver oils; milk, butter, cheese, eggs; can be manufactured by the body from carotene, a substance found in carrots, tomatoes, and the outer skin of green vegetables.	Vitamin A protects the body from infection and contributes to the processes of growth. A lack of it leads to diseases of the eye. It is possible to take too much vitamin A. Professional workers in child health clinics are alert for symptoms of overdosage.
B vitamins	Unrefined cereals, liver, yeast, nuts, some meat and Marmite.	This very complex group of vitamins has several different components. Lack of any one of them leads to diseases of the skin or nervous system, and is also thought to cause some types of mental confusion.

Nutrient	In which foods	Importance to body
Vitamin C	Fresh citrus fruits, early summer fruits such as strawberries, potatoes and some green vegetables such as the outer leaves of cabbage.	Vitamin C aids the body's healing power. It cannot be stored in the body so must be taken daily. Without it a condition known as scurvy arises, which can prove fatal if not recognized and treated. Although obvious cases of scurvy are rare, a number of elderly people who live on a diet of tea, bread and butter do suffer from a mild degree of the disease.
Vitamin D	Eggs, fish liver oils; can be made by the body when the skin is exposed to sunlight, although this source is only reliable in certain countries.	Vitamin D is essential for the proper use of calcium and phosphorus in the body; lack of it leads to a disease of the bone known as rickets. It is possible to have too much of this vitamin; parents who give their children cod or halibut liver oil should not exceed the stated dose. Workers in health clinics are alert for symptoms of overdosage.
Vitamin E	Wheatgerm, milk, cereals, egg yolk, liver.	Vitamin E helps to prevent cells from damage and degeneration.
Mineral salts (especially iron)	Eggs, cocoa, liver and baked beans; in some cases of iron-deficiency anaemia the doctor may prescribe iron tablets. Remember to keep these tablets in a safe place: they are brightly coloured and look like sweets but are highly dangerous to young children. If enough are taken, they can be fatal.	The body needs small quantities of mineral salts to maintain its functions and in a well-balanced diet there are enough of these. Iron, however, vital for the formation of red blood cells, is often in short supply. If the body has insufficient iron a condition known as iron-deficiency anaemia results. This is common, especially in pregnant women.
Water	Water is taken in when liquids are drunk and when food is eaten, since many foods contain a high proportion of water.	Water is vital to life. The body is 70 per cent water: nearly all body tissues contain water and many glands produce quite large quantities of watery secretions. Water is constantly being lost from the body: through the skin, the air breathed out and the elimination of water and faeces. Many people do not realize how essential fluid is and do not drink enough.

Food Habits

Although the diet of a healthy person must contain essential nutrients, these can be obtained in many ways and there are no essential foods. Even in a small country like Britain, food patterns vary from one part of the country to another: high tea is more popular in the north of England than the south, for instance. It should not therefore be surprising that the food habits of people in other countries are often very different. Many French enjoy frogs legs and snails. More extreme still, snakes and maggots are regarded as delicacies by certain Australian aborigines and spiders are eaten by some American Indians.

Food habits are established in childhood and familiar food gives a sense of security. Some men are so rigid in their habits that they will only eat food prepared by their mother or their wife. Others are reluctant to try new dishes when abroad, even though most people accept unfamiliar food as part of the enjoyment of a holiday. For the same reasons, immigrants often find it difficult to adopt the food patterns of their new country. Religious beliefs may play as large a part in this as traditional attitudes.

A little knowledge of your patient's food habits will help you when preparing a meal. The Moslem is forbidden alcohol and pork, but other types of meat are acceptable provided that they have been ritually killed. Orthodox Jews have rigid food laws: meat and fowl must be killed by specialists and prepared according to Jewish laws so as to become kosher or ritually fit to eat. Pork, bacon, ham, rabbit and shellfish are forbidden and meat and milk may not be eaten at the same meal. The Hindu is not allowed to eat beef. The vegetarian never eats meat, fish, dripping, fish oils, gelatine, rennet or suet (anything in fact that necessitates killing an animal) but he will eat dairy products. A vegan is a very strict vegetarian who will not even take dairy products and relies on milk, butter and cheese made from nuts or soya.

Helping the Patient to Eat

A meal should be as enjoyable an occasion as possible. It is all the more pleasurable if eaten in agreeable surroundings at a well appointed table. This applies to the sick person no less than it does to the healthy one.

The Patient Who Can Feed Himself

The patient must be comfortable. Give him the opportunity to empty his bladder and wash his hands before the meal. Make sure he is warm and well supported with pillows. When you bring the tray, make sure it is clean and set with all the requirements. The patient will find it irritating to watch his meal get cold while you run for the salt you forgot to put on the tray. The food itself should be prepared to give the maximum enjoyment, especially if the patient needs tempting to eat. Serve it in small portions and garnish it to make it look attractive and colourful. Give the patient time to eat each course but, as soon as he has finished the meal, remove the tray from the bedroom.

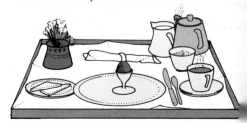

The Blind Patient

The blind patient is often able to feed himself with encouragement and a little thoughtful preparation, so be careful not to limit his independence. Cut the food up into bite-sized pieces and arrange it around the plate. You can then tell him that the potatoes are at 1 o'clock, the meat at 4 o'clock and so on. If he cannot feed himself, try and avoid saying "next" or "open" when each mouthful is ready; instead tap his chin when you want him to open his mouth. This leaves you free to chat.

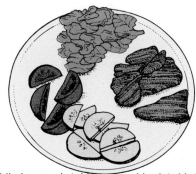

If a blind person is told where on his plate his food is, he can select balanced mouthfuls for himself.

The Patient without Teeth

The patient without natural teeth may find chewing difficult and need a soft diet. When preparing food you may find a mincer, liquidizer or emulsifier useful. Avoid extra spices and seasoning as healed gum surfaces are very sensitive.

The Helpless Patient

Some patients are in the unenviable position of being unable to feed themselves, so you must undertake this important task. Before the meal, help the patient into a comfortable position and protect the bedclothes with a napkin. Bring the tray to the bedside just as you would to any other patient, as the sight and smell of food can still give pleasure and increase appetite. Find out the patient's preferences regarding temperature and flavour.

Sit down by the patient and feed him with a fork or a spoon, allowing time for each mouthful to be properly chewed. Give drinks from a feeding cup (see page 65). Turn each mealtime into a pleasure.

When you are feeding a helpless patient, you may chat to her while she eats. Do not, however, force her to talk back to you throughout the meal.

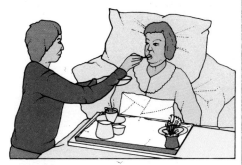

The Unconscious Patient

When a patient is unconscious, the swallowing reflex is lost. Any food or fluid put into the mouth is likely to drain down into the lungs, perhaps causing death from asphyxiation. This is why it is so important not to try and give an unconscious or even semi-conscious person a drink — it may prove fatal. Such patients are fed either by a tube through the mouth and into the stomach or by special sterile fluids into a vein. You are unlikely to have to feed an unconscious patient.

Helping to Prepare Meals

The elderly, arthritic and disabled often find preparing meals difficult. Physical handicaps may be relieved by the provision of various kitchen aids but, in some cases, regularly prepared meals can be provided.

You may also come into contact with the patient living on his own who cannot be bothered to cook for himself. He may just need encouragement and company or he may also need regularly prepared meals.

Meals on Wheels

The Meals on Wheels service provides a regular midday meal. Ideally the service runs from Monday to Friday but, in some cases, a meal is provided two or three times a week. The service is run by the Women's Royal Voluntary Service or other voluntary services as agents for the Social Services Department. Clients pay a fixed contribution each time a meal is delivered.

Aids to Eating and Drinking

Many aids exist to help people with different types of disability, ranging from weakness in the hands to loss of the use of one arm. Most of the aids illustrated here are designed to encourage independence among patients; some, the feeding cups, are intended for use with helpless patients. (Note: the patient drinks the fluid at the bottom of the feeding cup first; make sure there are no tea leaves or coffee grounds in the drink.)

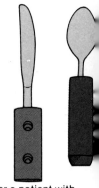

For a patient with arthritic hands, light but thick-handled cutlery (above) is easier to grasp. It can be bought in a variety of different designs or improvised by padding ordinary cutlery with foam rubber.

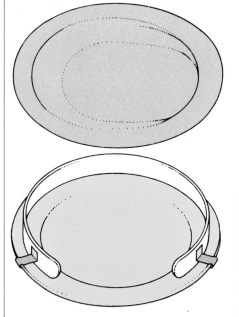

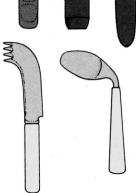

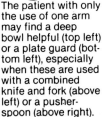

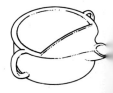

The patient with only the use of one arm may find a deep bowl helpful (top left) or a plate guard (bottom left), especially when these are used with a combined knife and fork (above left) or a pusher-spoon (above right).

the amount varies according to the locality. Although the service's main function is to provide a meal, it also means each client is seen daily or at regular intervals by a volunteer who is interested in his welfare. As a general rule, the Meals on Wheels service does not cater for special diets.

Day centres and clubs

Day centres and luncheon clubs are usually run by the statutory authorities and by voluntary groups. Many provide a mid-day meal for those attending the centre for the day, while luncheon clubs often cater only for the midday meal. For more about day centres see page 141.

Marie Curie Foundation

Patients with some form of cancer may be eligible for special help from the Marie Curie Foundation. For instance, if the patient has difficulty in swallowing, the Foundation may fund the purchase of special food and equipment such as a liquidizer. If there is anything the patient needs, talk to the district nursing sister.

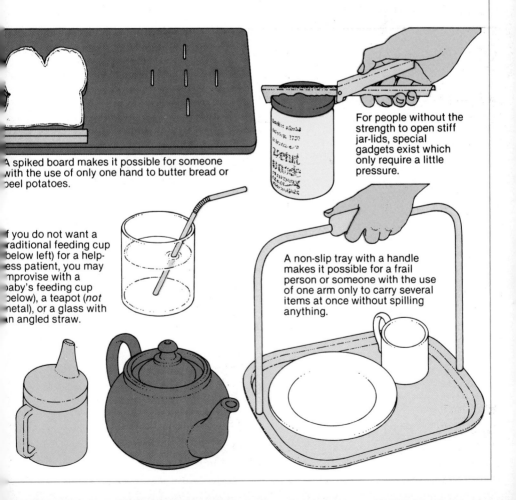

A spiked board makes it possible for someone with the use of only one hand to butter bread or peel potatoes.

For people without the strength to open stiff jar-lids, special gadgets exist which only require a little pressure.

If you do not want a traditional feeding cup (below left) for a help-less patient, you may improvise with a baby's feeding cup (below), a teapot (*not* metal), or a glass with an angled straw.

A non-slip tray with a handle makes it possible for a frail person or someone with the use of one arm only to carry several items at once without spilling anything.

Minor Digestive Problems

Many patients confined to bed for much of the time suffer from heartburn or indigestion, while occasional vomiting is a part of several different conditions.

Heartburn and Indigestion

Heartburn and indigestion are two very common problems, which cause a large amount of discomfort. Heartburn is caused by the back flow of stomach acid into the oesophagus. It is felt as a burning sensation in the centre of the chest (hence its name "heartburn"). The sufferer often feels most uncomfortable after a large meal, when he is lying down or bending over to pick something up from the floor.

Indigestion is most commonly the result of unwise eating. Rich or spicy foods, excessive alcohol or smoking can all cause a temporary inflammation of the stomach lining. The patient has a sensation of fullness and discomfort in the upper abdomen, sometimes with belching and nausea.

The best way of preventing heartburn and indigestion is to avoid giving the patient large, rich or spicy meals. Alcohol should be taken in moderation and not on an empty stomach. Smoking should be restricted.

The acid in the stomach can be neutralized with a glass of milk or a mild antacid tablet. Warm milk is particularly effective at night. Sit the patient up if the discomfort is severe. Do not give a strong antacid (or any antacid over a long period) without the doctor's consent. If the patient is suffering from a great deal of flatulence, peppermint water sipped slowly is very effective. If pain persists or recurs, inform the district nursing sister or the doctor.

Vomiting

Vomiting is distressing for the patient, especially if it happens without warning.

If a patient starts to vomit, fetch a bowl immediately. Remove any false teeth if you can. Steady the bowl. If the bedclothes have soiled, cover them with a paper towel while the attack lasts. When it is over give the patient a mouthwash and wash his face and hands, before changing his bed-linen and clothing as necessary.

Observe the amount and character of the vomit. Unless it is either water or undigested food, save a specimen for the doctor. Place this in a covered jar and keep it in a cool place away from the patient. Observe his colour and pulse rate. Make a note of:
- the time of vomiting
- whether the vomiting is associated with eating or drinking
- whether pain is associated with the vomiting (in some conditions pain is relieved by vomiting; in others it increases).

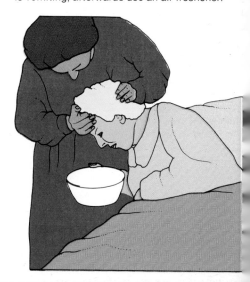

Support the patient's head over a bowl while she is vomiting; afterwards use an air freshener.

Feeding the New Baby

Deciding whether to breast or bottle-feed is one of the major decisions every new mother has to make and most mothers — particularly with their first baby — will want advice. This should be readily available from someone with knowledge and experience, such as the midwife or health visitor.

The wishes of the mother are as important as the needs of the baby. Whatever method is adopted, satisfactory infant feeding depends on a contented baby and a happy mother.

Breast-Feeding

Breast milk looks rather like water. It is quite different from cow's milk. Many mothers think that their milk is "no good for the baby" because it looks so watery. This is not the case: breast milk is meant to look exactly the way it does. It also contains valuable antibodies. As long as the mother is eating well, the baby will receive all he needs for the first months of life.

Breast-feeding is easier than bottle-feeding. The milk does not need to be sterilized, nor does it need to be warmed. It does not have to be specially stored, nor does it have to be prepared before use.

When to feed

Many mothers prefer the idea of fixed feeding times. During the first weeks of the baby's life, however, they will be lucky and unusual if their baby also prefers fixed feeding times! Demand feeding usually turns out to be more satisfactory for both mother and baby. Instead of keeping a crying baby waiting for his next feed, or waking a sleeping baby when it is "time" to feed him, the baby is fed when he is hungry.

In fact, babies who are on a self-demand schedule usually acquire a routine of their own. Feeding times will rarely be evenly spaced but will nevertheless be found to occur at about the same time every day.

All babies need feeding at night for at least their first six weeks of life. Some persist in wanting an extra night feed for weeks or even months. In these circumstances, patience is the only solution. The baby will not go on wanting to be fed at 2am or 3am for ever; in the meantime it would be unfair to refuse his demand.

Positions for feeding

A comfortable position, plenty of time and — especially in the first weeks — all the privacy you need are the basic requirements for giving satisfactory feeds. You should hold the baby so that his head is supported well above the level of his stomach.

The ideal chair for nursing is low, upright and armless. It provides good support for your back, as long as the baby is correctly positioned for you — perhaps with the help of a pillow.

If you choose to feed your baby lying down, make sure that most of your weight is taken by pillows. You will soon feel tired if you spend the feed leaning on your elbow.

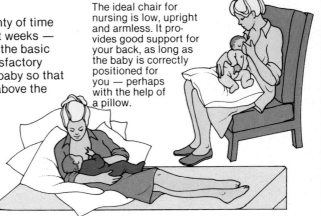

How much to give

There is no accurate way of telling how much milk a baby takes when he is breast-fed. For some mothers, this uncertainty is one of the strongest inducements to bottle-feed. If, however, a mother can be persuaded to continue with breast-feeding, within a very short period of time she will know well enough whether or not her baby is satisfied.

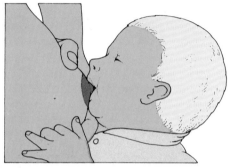

The baby should feed with both the nipple and the surrounding area in his mouth for the best flow of milk. Make sure he has room to breathe while he sucks.

How long to take

Feeding time is not merely an opportunity to get food into the baby. Mother and baby need to get to know each other and to build up the ties that come from the physical contact of feeding.

As a general rule, about ten minutes sucking at each breast is adequate, and it is customary to start on alternate sides at each feed. Some babies get all they want from one breast, others need only five minutes on each side. Others still are only content if they are allowed twenty minutes or more at each breast. A mother soon learns to know when her baby has had enough.

Wind and colic

Whether breast or bottle-fed, most babies get wind. This is because their sucking is not completely efficient and some air is gulped in with the milk. Usually mothers find it best to pause halfway through a feed, take the baby from the breast, and place him against her shoulder or upright on her lap while gently patting his back.

Babies who cry frequently, apparently from some kind of pain in the abdomen, have rarely just got wind. In most instances the baby has colic and expert advice is needed. Some babies cry regularly between the 6pm and 10pm feeds every evening. This can be very disturbing for both parents. However, it usually stops spontaneously when the baby is about 13 weeks old, and has thus been given the name "three-month colic". What causes it is not clear, nor why it happens in the early evening. Time usually improves matters without other help.

Alleviating mothers' anxieties

Many mothers want to breast-feed, but feel that their supply is inadequate. In the first few days after birth this is quite normal. After that Nature usually achieves a perfect balance between the demands of the baby and the mother's ability to satisfy him.

There are no specific foods or fluids which will improve the supply of milk. Neither are there any special medicines which are known to help. A mother who really feels worried that her baby is not thriving because she has not got enough milk should take expert advice.

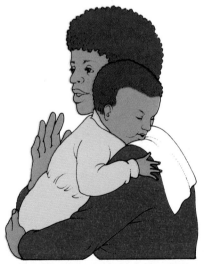

Some babies bring up a little milk along with air when they burp. This is quite normal, but a sensible mother usually protects her clothing.

Bottle-Feeding

If a mother is really unhappy at the prospect of breast-feeding her child, or if in exceptional circumstances she proves unable to do so, bottle-feeding is a perfectly adequate and acceptable alternative.

Choice of bottle and teat

Feeding bottles can be made either of glass or of plastic. For convenience measurements of volume are marked on the side.

The shape of the sucking end of the teat resembles the human nipple as nearly as possible. The teat should have a hole large enough to allow milk to drip out unaided when the bottle is held upside down, at a rate of several drops a second. If an existing hole is too small, it can be enlarged by piercing the teat with a red-hot needle (placing the eye of the needle in a cork before heating it will prevent burnt fingers). Sterilize the teat before use (see below).

Choice of foods

There are many varieties of milk on the market that are suitable for feeding babies — and a few that are not. Giving unmodified milks to babies under six months old is dangerous.

The usual substitute for breast milk is cow's milk in one form or another. The best types to use are proprietary milk powders intended for babies. These may be bought at chemists' shops. Most child health clinics also sell branded dried milks, usually in cardboard packets, at a reduced price. There is no significant difference between any of the standard dried milks: they have all been modified to resemble breast milk as closely as possible.

Sterilizing feeding equipment

In preparing any type of food for a baby, contamination with germs must be avoided. All utensils used must be sterilized and you should wash your hands before you start.

Immediately after use all bottles and teats should be rinsed inside and out with

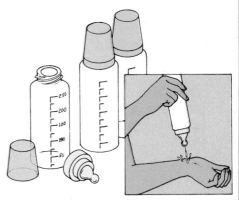

The number of bottles you have will depend on how you organize your sterilizing. Even if you are breast-feeding you will need one or two bottles for giving water or juice. Milk should flow from the teats at the rate of several drops a second.

cold water, washed in warm water with washing-up liquid, then rinsed again. The teat should be rubbed inside with salt and rinsed once more. Bottles and teats should then be immersed in a container filled with sterile solution. It is important that no air bubbles are trapped inside the bottles or teats. If you have not bought a purpose-made container, you may need to cover the teats with a glass to stop them floating to the top. Leave the bottles and teats in the solution for at least two hours before draining. Do not rinse before re-using.

It is also possible to sterilize feeding equipment by placing it in a large saucepan of warm water and boiling the equipment for three minutes.

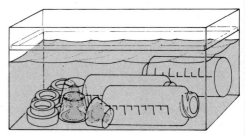

Everything in a container of sterile solution must be completely submerged if it is to be effectively sterilized.

Preparing bottle-feeds

Before you start, clear a working surface or spread out a clean towel. Collect everything you need, making sure that all bottles and teats are sterile. Wash your hands. Follow exactly the instruction on the packet or tin of formula you are using. If in doubt, check with the midwife or health visitor.

Many mothers find it convenient to make up a day's supply of bottles at once and store them in the refrigerator.

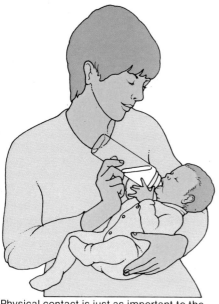

Physical contact is just as important to the bottle-fed baby as to the breast-fed one. Make sure the teat is full of milk, not air.

How to give a bottle-feed

Place the bottle with its teat and cover in a jug of hot water. Wash your hands and sit in a comfortable chair. Support the baby just as if you were breast-feeding (see page 68). Before giving the feed shake a little milk on to the back of your hand: it should be comfortably warm, not hot.

The aim of bottle-feeding is to make it as like breast-feeding as possible. The same relationship needs to be established between mother and baby and the mother should therefore be encouraged to feed the baby herself whenever possible.

Weaning

The addition of solids to a baby's diet is called "weaning" and is usually begun at about four months and completed by nine months. Only very small amounts are given at first to introduce new flavours, prevent digestive upsets, and get the baby used to the idea of solid food.

The kind of food given depends on whether or not the baby can chew. Most babies begin to chew at about six months, even if they have not yet got any teeth. Before the baby can chew he must be given foods which can be swallowed as they are. These could be pre-cooked baby cereals, fruit and vegetable puree, gravy (especially from fresh meat), grated cheese, egg yolk, mashed banana and even very finely minced meat. There are many proprietary baby foods and cereals on the market and these are quick and easy to use, but where possible fresh foods are preferable.

Each food must be introduced in a small amount. A teaspoonful twice a day is adequate at first and if the baby refuses that particular food it should not be offered again for several days. Similarly the stools should be observed for signs of digestive upsets.

Once the baby can chew, the variety of foods can be increased. By his second year he will be able to have almost anything that is being served at a family meal.

Feeding the sick child

What a child eats when he is ill should be regulated by his appetite. Fluids are important, especially if he is vomiting or has diarrhoea. Clear fluids are best, such as water, plain or flavoured. Milk may make vomiting worse and is not advisable for babies with diarrhoea.

In short illnesses of a week or less there is no need to encourage the appetite with specially prepared tit-bits. A small helping of a child's normal diet will be acceptable. On the other hand, in a prolonged illness the patient should be encouraged to take foods essential for growth, health, and repair to diseased tissue: that is, a diet rich in proteins and vitamins (see page 62).

GIVING MEDICINES:
Helping the patient to take and care for his medicines

GIVING MEDICINES

The ancients were studying simple plants for their healing properties long before anything precise was known about the nature of drugs. The plants were used to prevent disease, cure illness or relieve symptoms, but nothing was known about their mode of action.

It is only in recent years that the study of drugs has developed into a highly exact science. The simple plants have been analysed and their active principles have been found. Research workers have found ways of producing many of them synthetically, so reducing their cost and increasing their purity. The number of drugs has increased, and the action of many is exceedingly powerful — so much so that there is now a range of diseases caused by the drugs themselves. Many drugs have side-effects: examples are the drowsiness that results from taking a sea-sickness pill or the weight gain that sometimes comes from taking the contraceptive pill.

Because of their potency and the possibility of side-effects which might be harmful, it is vital that drugs are given only to the person for whom the doctor prescribed them. No patient should ever be allowed to use up a drug originally prescribed for somebody else.

If you are looking after a patient in the home, you may be called upon to give him medicines. Medicines may contain one or more drugs. As long as you exercise due care, give only what the doctor ordered, and follow four basic rules, errors should not occur.

These are the four basic rules:
1 Check the medicine to make sure it is the right one
2 Give the exact amount ordered
3 Give it to the patient for whom it was prescribed
4 Give it at the time ordered by the doctor.

If you want to remember these four rules easily and quickly, think of them as giving:
- the right amount
- of the right medicine
- to the right patient
- at the right time.

Medicines by Mouth

The most usual way of giving drugs is by mouth. Medicines given by mouth come in several forms. They may be liquids, tablets, capsules, pills or powders. You will proceed slightly differently according to the type of drug you are giving.

Before you start to give any type of drug, prepare a small tray. On it should be a glass of water, the drugs you need, and a medicine glass or spoon. Many medicines are now supplied with a 5ml spoon for convenience.

Giving Tablets, Capsules or Pills

You must first check the bottle by reading the label. Shake out the correct number of tablets into a spoon and read the label again. Give the tablet to the patient in the spoon, accompanied by a glass of water. Make sure he swallows the tablet. Some tablets are very large and may be difficult to swallow. Tablets can usually be divided into smaller pieces with a knife, although it is not possible to divide capsules and pills.

If the patient finds swallowing tablets difficult, crush them up between metal spoons so that he can either swallow the powder with water, or take it in a spoonful of jam or honey.

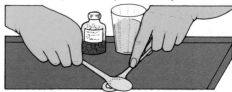

Giving Liquids

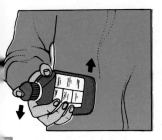 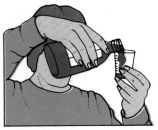 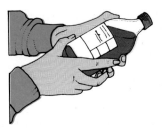

1 Check the bottle by reading the label. Place a finger over the cork or screwtop and shake the bottle several times. Remove the top and hold it with your little finger.

2 Hold the bottle label uppermost, so that, when pouring, any drips will not obliterate the instructions. Hold the glass **at eye level** and accurately measure the dose ordered.

3 Replace the cork or screwtop and read the label again. Give the dose to the patient and make sure he drinks it. Offer water afterwards. Wipe the bottle and wash the glass or spoon.

Giving Powders

You can either mix the powder with jam or honey or stir it into a small quantity of milk or water and give it to the patient at once.

Remember that if the patient is being given a special diet, any jam or honey should be considered as part of that diet.

Drugs: Rectum

Drugs given this way are given as suppositories or retention enemas. They are inserted into the rectum and the patient is asked to try and retain them. The drug is absorbed slowly and the effect lasts for several hours. See page 83 for more about how suppositories and enemas are given.

Inhalation

Drugs given this way are added to steam and take the form of an inhalation (see page 125). Alternatively the patient may be provided with an aerosol containing the relevant drug, which he can use for himself when he needs to. Such drugs are intended to relieve breathing in conditions such as asthma or bronchitis.

Injection

Injections will normally be given by the doctor or professional nurse, but you should know that there are various types of injection. Subcutaneous injections are injected just under the skin; intramuscular are injected rather deeper into muscle; intravenous are injected into a vein.

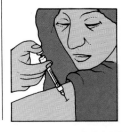

A diabetic patient needing to have regular injections will be taught how to inject herself by a professional nurse. Parents of diabetic children may also be taught how to give the necessary injections.

Drops

Drops may be applied to the eye, ear or nose. They are supplied in small bottles fitted with droppers, in little plastic containers or even as a single application. Some are dangerous if taken by mouth, so keep them away from children.

Administering Eye Drops

Check if the drops are to go into one or both eyes. This is important: many eye drops are prescribed for a specific eye and they may cause serious damage or even blindness if put into the other eye by mistake. Ask the patient to sit down and wash your hands. Stand behind him and ask him to look up. Hold the dropper horizontally, with your hand resting on his face. Apply slight pressure to the lower eyelid to bring it away from the eyeball and insert the drop gently into this space. Let the eye close and ask the patient to blink. This spreads the drop over the whole surface of the eye.

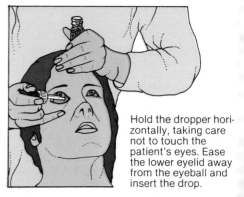

Hold the dropper horizontally, taking care not to touch the patient's eyes. Ease the lower eyelid away from the eyeball and insert the drop.

Administering Ear Drops

Warm the drops by standing the container in a bowl of warm water. Protect the patient's clothing with a small paper towel and wash your hands. Ask him either to lie down with the affected ear uppermost, or to sit with his head tilted so that the affected ear is uppermost. Rest the tip of the dropper just above the ear and allow the drops to trickle down into it. Ask the patient to keep his head in the same position for a few minutes.

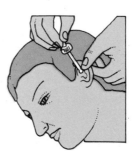

Make sure that the patient's head is tilted with the affected ear uppermost. With the tip of the dropper resting just above the ear, let the drops ooze gently in. The patient should not move his head for a few minutes after the drops have been inserted.

Administering Nasal Drops

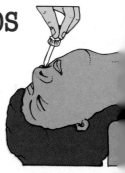

Wash your hands. Lay the patient down on his back so that his head is hanging over the edge of the bed. Alternatively, sit him down and tilt his head back as far as possible. Wash your hands. Insert the tip of the dropper just inside the nostril and allow a drop to go in. Repeat on the other side. Ask the patient to sniff. If he is lying across the bed, leave him there for a few minutes.

Ideally the patient should receive nasal drops lying across a bed on his back with his head hanging down over the edge. This position, however, is uncomfortable. He may therefore prefer to sit down and tilt his head well back.

Care and Custody of Medicines

Most accidents connected with drugs occur in the home because of carelessness. In hospitals and institutions stringent rules exist for the care and custody of drugs.

Storing Medicines

If you abide by the following rules, drugs will be safe in your care.
● keep drugs for internal use in a safe place, apart from substances intended for external application
● never transfer medicines from their original bottles to other containers
● never mix different sorts of pills and tablets in the same container
● keep medicines in a cool place: the doctor will tell you if any drug needs to be stored in a refrigerator
● do not use any medicine if you cannot read its label clearly.

Deterioration of Medicines

Drugs deteriorate and it is necessary to be able to recognize substances unfit for use.
● do not give drugs or drops that have passed their expiry date
● do not give any substance, liquid or solid, that has changed colour
● do not give an originally clear liquid that has become cloudy or has developed a sediment that was not there before
● do not give if you cannot read the label
● do not give a drug if anything raises a doubt in your mind about giving it.

Disposing of Medicines

When a drug is no longer required it should be flushed down the lavatory. If a patient has died, dispose of drugs he was taking.

If a disposable syringe has been used to give an injection, replace the cover and snap off the nozzle. Wrap the syringe and the needle in newspaper before placing it in a dustbin. This will prevent the refuse collector from being injured and drug addicts from getting hold of a used syringe.

Categories of medicine

Drugs fall into several categories: general sale medicines that can be bought in any shop or supermarket; pharmacy medicines which can only be sold under the supervision of a pharmacist; drugs obtainable on prescription only.

Among the substances obtainable on prescription from a doctor only are the controlled drugs. These are substances which make the taker dependent on them. This group includes strong pain-killers such as opium, morphine and heroin; sleeping tablets such as barbiturates; and stimulants such as amphetamines. All are taken "for kicks" by drug addicts.

Stringent legislation controls the ordering, storage and use of these drugs in hospital. If you are undertaking hospital duties, you must make yourself familiar with hospital rulings.

In the home, if a patient of yours is taking controlled drugs, your responsibility is to ensure that the drugs are stored in a safe place. If they are tablets, check how many are left each time a dose is given to the patient.

Giving Medicines to Children

If medicines have been prescribed for a child by a doctor, the child needs those medicines. He should take them, even if he dislikes them or if he seems better.

Most children take their medicine quite readily. Liquid medicines are often prescribed for small children, in which case you should have a glass of the child's favourite drink ready to wash the taste of the medicine away after he has taken it. If the child really dislikes the taste of his medicine, you can disguise the taste by mixing the medicine with a spoonful of jam or honey. Do not pretend to the child that you are only giving him jam: he will notice the drug and will not trust you again. Tell him that it is medicine but that it will not taste unpleasant this way.

Keeping medicines safe

It is important not to confuse medicines with sweets for another reason: the child may get the idea that all pills are nice to eat, especially if he has been used to taking sugar-coated coloured pills. Many iron pills, for instance, are perfectly safe in the recommended dose, but they look like chocolate buttons and children may swallow them in handfuls.

Every medicine should be regarded as potentially dangerous to children. Some are more dangerous than others, but no tablets are completely safe if too many are swallowed. For this reason medicines should not be kept within reach of small fingers. They should be locked in a safe cupboard with the key kept somewhere different, not left in the door. Medicines to be kept in the cupboard should include *all* substances containing drugs: skin creams and menthol for inhalation, not just liquids and pills.

Special safety bottles with "childproof" tops can be purchased. If medicines are always kept in a locked cupboard, safety tops are not strictly speaking necessary, but there is never any harm in taking extra precautions.

In any normal household there are many ordinary products which are also potentially dangerous. Experience has shown that the following are particularly hazardous: ammonia; antifreeze liquid; brake fluid; caustic soda; oven cleaner; paintbrush restorer; paint stripper. It is better to be safe than sorry. Keep these substances and any others that are similarly not intended for internal use under lock and key, *not* in the cupboard under the kitchen sink.

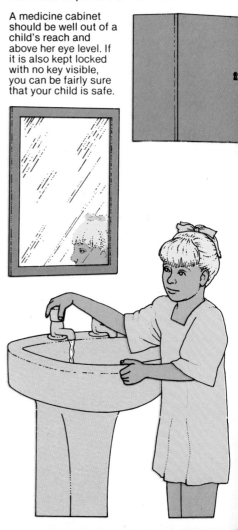

A medicine cabinet should be well out of a child's reach and above her eye level. If it is also kept locked with no key visible, you can be fairly sure that your child is safe.

ELIMINATION:
Helping the patient to deal
with his excretions

ELIMINATION

Helping the patient with elimination is one of the most testing aspects of your nursing care. A difficult and embarrassing service for the patient to accept, he must never sense that it is difficult or embarrassing for you to give. Your priority is to maintain the patient's dignity at all times, even if he is unconscious, and to provide privacy whenever possible.

The normal elimination from the body is from the bladder, the bowel and the skin. Women regularly lose menstrual fluid from the vagina. When people are ill they may vomit (see page 66) or have a cough and produce sputum (see page 128). All these excretions are often saved, as they may provide valuable information about the patient's condition.

Menstrual fluid

Most female patients of childbearing age continue to menstruate when they are ill. You will need to see that a supply of sanitary pads, along with a belt or protective pads, is available, or tampons if preferred. If the patient is not allowed out of bed she may find it difficult or impossible to insert a tampon, so pads may have to be used.

Every time a bedpan or commode is used, provide a paper bag for the soiled sanitary pad. If the sheets get stained the patient may be extremely embarrassed. Change them with the minimum of fuss and soak them in cold water or a biological detergent.

The patient may suffer pain (dysmenorrhoea), particularly if she is normally active. A well-protected hot water bottle (see page 102) and a mild pain-killer (analgesic) if allowed will usually be adequate treatment.

Basic Care

To attend to the patient's needs satisfactorily, you must know how much he is able to do for himself and have some idea of the times when he is likely to need help. He may be able to walk to the lavatory, perhaps with just a steadying hand from you; but he may not be able to go as far as the lavatory, in which case he may either be allowed out of bed in the bedroom to use a commode or have to use a bedpan or urinal in bed.

The patient must be given the opportunity to follow his usual habits. Most people tend to pass urine soon after they get up in the morning and many have been in the habit from childhood of passing urine before a meal and last thing before going to sleep at night.

Using a Commode

Make sure the bedroom door is closed before helping the patient out of bed. Put his slippers on for him and place a dressing gown or shawl around his shoulders. If necessary help the patient to move his pyjamas or her nightdress out of the way, and seat him carefully. Cover him with a blanket: this muffles the sound of the urine and reduces embarrassment, both from the sound and from exposure. See that there is a toilet roll within the patient's reach and leave him in peace — unless he is weak or unsteady, in which case remain nearby. Afterwards encourage him to wash his hands; if it is not possible for him to walk as far as the nearest basin, have ready a bowl of water, soap and a towel for his immediate use.

Giving a Bedpan

Make sure the bedpan is warm and dry before taking it to the bedside covered with a paper towel or piece of kitchen roll. Also take a toilet roll. Make sure the bedroom door is closed to ensure privacy. Help the patient to lift up her nightdress or slide down his pyjama trousers. Use one hand to help him raise himself while you slip the pan under him with the other. (If he is allowed to sit upright against pillows, the whole procedure is easier and more natural.) After he has finished, let him use the toilet paper, unless he is too ill to manage when you will need to attend to this for him. Take the pan away from him and cover it immediately. Re-arrange the nightclothes and bedlinen and make the patient comfortable. This is often a good opportunity for changing his position in bed, so helping to prevent pressure sores (see p. 29).

Let the patient wash his hands while you take the covered pan to the lavatory and rinse it with cold water. Wash your own hands.

Male patients will only require a bedpan for a bowel action. They should be given a urinal at the same time, as well as when they may need to pass urine.

Giving a Urinal

Cover the urinal with a paper towel or a piece of kitchen roll, take it to the bedside and hand it to the patient. If he is very ill or helpless, place it in position. After use, cover it, empty it and rinse it in cold water.

Many men have difficulty in passing urine lying down; whenever possible they should be allowed to stand by the bedside. If a urinal is not available, a wide-mouthed jar is a good substitute.

Aids in the Lavatory

Various aids exist to help the elderly and disabled to use the lavatory by themselves.

They may be of great help to frail, arthritic, paralysed or elderly people.

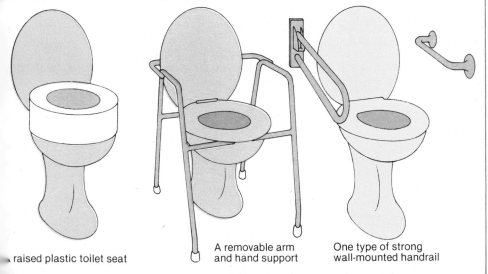

A raised plastic toilet seat

A removable arm and hand support

One type of strong wall-mounted handrail

Urine

The two kidneys filter the blood and produce urine from the waste products extracted. The urine passes down two tubes, the ureters, into the bladder. As the bladder fills it stretches, and nerve impulses are communicated to the brain signalling that the bladder is full and must be emptied. The urine is then passed from the urethra, a small tube connecting the bladder to the body surface.

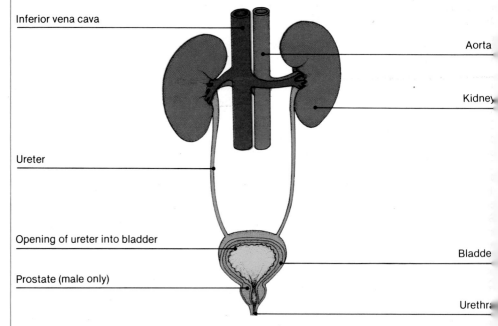

Inferior vena cava

Aorta

Kidney

Ureter

Opening of ureter into bladder

Bladder

Prostate (male only)

Urethra

Saving a Specimen

To save a specimen of urine, collect it in a clean, dry bedpan or urinal. Pour some into a clean, dry bottle or jar, which you either cork or screw tightly. Label the bottle with the patient's full name and address, the date and time of collection and the nature of the specimen.

You may be asked to save specimens of urine over a 24-hour period. On the appointed day when the patient first empties his bladder, discard the urine. After that, each time the patient passes urine in the course of the day, put it into a polythene or glass jar or bottle with a stopper or suitable cover. The last specimen to go into the jar is the urine first passed by the patient the following day. Again you should label the jar with the patient's name and address, the date of collection and the nature of the specimen.

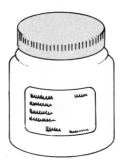

A urine specimen may be collected in any clean bottle or jar as long as it is clearly labelled. If you are given a container by a doctor or hospital, it may resemble the one shown here.

Measuring Output

t is sometimes necessary to know exactly how much urine the patient is passing. A jug that measures fluid in millilitres or ounces should be kept in the lavatory for this purpose. The patient can pass urine into the jug or you can pour urine from a bedpan or urinal into the jug. Note the quantity of urine and write this down, together with a record of the time the urine was passed. Every day at the same time, total and record the quantity. As the urinary output is influenced by the amount the patient drinks, the intake is also often measured and recorded.

Urine Testing

In illness there may be obvious changes in the urine and these should be carefully noticed.

Colour: Urine is normally yellow, but it may become dark if it is concentrated, or much paler if the patient is drinking a great deal. Certain drugs may also alter the colour.

Appearance: Normally urine is clear, but the presence of abnormalities may make it cloudy.

Smell: Some infections or drugs (for instance, antibiotics) may cause urine to have a distinct odour. If it is left in contact with the air for any length of time it smells of ammonia.

Quantity: Normally a person passes about 500 ml of urine a day, although this quantity is affected by the amount of fluid drunk. In some illnesses, the patient may pass very small quantities of urine and in extreme cases none at all. This is a grave sign, which must be reported immediately. On the other hand, in some diseases the output of urine is increased; the patient feels thirsty and drinks extra fluid.

Frequency: In certain conditions urine is passed at abnormally frequent intervals and may disturb the patient's rest at night. This should be reported.

Pain: The patient may feel pain on passing urine or discomfort before starting to pass urine. If this is the case the doctor should be informed.

If any abnormality in the urine is observed or suspected, report this to the doctor and save a specimen for him.

It is possible to discover the presence of abnormalities in the urine by chemical tests. These tests were once very complicated but are now simple. In normal circumstances it is unlikely that you would be asked to test urine, but you may see it being tested by the doctor or nurse, or in some conditions by the patient.

The common abnormalities found in urine are protein, blood, sugar, acetone, bile and pus. If these substances come into contact with certain specific chemicals they react in a typical and obvious way, so that their presence can be confirmed. The chemicals are incorporated in small sticks of card and the testing is done by dipping the stick in the urine and watching to see if the stick changes colour. If the urine is acid, blue card will turn pink; if it is alkaline, pink card will turn blue; if neither card changes colour the urine is neutral.

Explicit instructions and colour charts are supplied with every set of sticks. As long as the instructions are carefully followed, the urine is tested simply, quickly and accurately.

Testing a baby's urine

The doctor might ask you to test a baby's urine if the napkin is dry when he calls. In these circumstances he will leave the necessary equipment: you will have a stick to press against a freshly wet (not merely a damp) napkin. You remove it immediately, wait for about half a minute; you then compare the colour of the stick with the colours on a chart and tell the doctor when he returns.

Faeces

The process of food digestion begins in the stomach, and is completed in the duodenum and small intestine. Nutrients are absorbed through the intestinal wall into the bloodstream. Water and undigested remains pass into the large intestine, where most of the water is reabsorbed. The remaining wastes, or faeces are expelled through the anal sphincter.

Normal stools are brown in colour and semisolid in consistency. Any deviation from the normal should be noted and a specimen saved for the doctor to see.

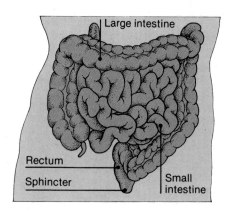

Saving a Specimen

If possible the patient should not pass urine at the same time as faeces when a specimen is to be collected. With men this is simple as urine is normally passed into a urinal. It is generally necessary to ask women to pass urine first, before emptying and washing the bedpan and bringing it back again.

Wear disposable plastic gloves if available Using a spatula, scoop some faeces into a waxed carton or screw-top jar. Label the container with the patient's full name and address, the date and time of collection, and the nature of the specimen. Wrap the gloves and spatula in newspaper before burning. Empty and clean the bedpan.

Diarrhoea

When a patient passes stools at frequent intervals he is said to have diarrhoea. The material passed becomes liquid and in severe cases may consist of coloured watery fluid. If diarrhoea persists, the patient suffers from loss of fluid or dehydration and may become very ill. Diarrhoea must always be reported to the doctor without delay. Diarrhoea is particularly serious in the baby or young child as dehydration occurs very rapidly and the baby can die in a matter of hours.

Constipation

The opposite of diarrhoea, constipation occurs when the bowel does not empty itself at its usual rhythm so the stools become dry and hard. Individual habits vary: some people normally pass two stools a day, while others may pass only one every 48 hours. Constipation occurs when the normal pattern is disturbed. **Constipation in the healthy person:** In an otherwise healthy person constipation may

be the result of not drinking enough fluid, not eating enough roughage or not allowing enough time for a bowel action. Roughage, which stimulates the bowel, is found in fresh fruit and vegetables, in cereals (especially unprocessed bran or porridge) and in wholemeal bread.

Correction of diet and habits will often relieve constipation. Medicines known as aperients are extensively advertised and widely used to speed up normal bowel movement and so cause an evacuation. They have no effect on the cause of constipation, however, and therefore the condition persists.

Constipation in the patient: When people are ill they often become constipated. This may be the result of restricted diet, of increased fluid loss from sweating, or simply of unaccustomed inactivity. The patient may also be reluctant to drink in an attempt to avoid bedpans.

Giving a suppository

A suppository is cone-shaped and contains a drug that causes the bowel to empty itself. Because it is made of a substance that melts at body temperature, it melts when placed in the rectum, but will also melt in the hand if held for too long.

Start by washing your hands and tell the patient what is to happen. See that he has passed urine before you begin. Help him to lie on his left side and draw up his knees. Ask him to relax by breathing deeply in and out through the mouth. Remove the foil from the suppository and put on a rubber glove or fingerstall. Dip the suppository in warm water before inserting it gently into the rectum and pushing it up as far as possible. If two have been ordered, insert the second in the same way. Remove the glove or fingerstall and place it in a paper bag before burning it or putting it in the dustbin. Wash your hands.

Encourage the patient to retain the sup-

Giving an enema

An enema is an injection of fluid into the rectum, usually given with the intention of stimulating a bowel movement. A disposable enema has the fluid contained in a small plastic bag and a rectal nozzle attached ready for use. Before use it should be warmed.

Start by washing your hands and tell the patient what is to happen. Help him to lie on his left side with his knees drawn up. See that he is adequately covered and place a paper towel on a piece of plastic under his buttocks to protect the bed. Ask him to relax by breathing in and out

You should assess the patient's condition and respond accordingly. Encourage him to drink more, unless for any reason fluids are restricted. Add fruit juice and roughage to the diet. Give him a bedpan or help him to the commode at a time when he would normally have a bowel movement. Above all, be sensitive to his feelings and his dignity: ensure his privacy and, if possible, leave him undisturbed.

If nothing else works the doctor may order a suppository or an enema.

pository for as long as possible before using the commode or bedpan. After a bowel action has taken place report on the stool, noting its colour, size and consistency.

Remember that some drugs are administered in the form of a suppository (see page 73); these are to be retained in the rectum so no bedpan should be given.

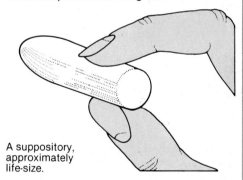

A suppository, approximately life-size.

through his mouth. Break off the tip of the nozzle and smear the nozzle with petroleum jelly. Insert it gently into the rectum for 8-10cm, taking care not to damage the rectal wall. Gently squeeze the bag, so injecting fluid into the rectum. Withdraw the nozzle into a paper tissue or kitchen paper.

Encourage the patient to retain the enema as long as possible before using the commode or bedpan. After a bowel action has taken place report on the stool, noting its colour, size and consistency. Wrap the enema apparatus in newspaper before burning it. Wash your hands.

Incontinence

Difficulty in the control of the bladder or bowel can occur at any age if there has been damage to the area or to the brain. The involuntary escape of urine or the emptying of the bowel is a very distressing and humiliating experience, and it is not surprising that people suffering from incontinence often tend to isolate themselves.

Urinary Incontinence

The bladder is a muscular bag, the outlet of which is guarded by two circular bands of muscle. A small baby has no control over this muscle and its bladder empties immediately and involuntarily. As we grow and the nerve pathways develop, we learn to control the muscle. From then on we are conscious when the bladder is full and have the control to wait for a convenient place before passing urine. It is when something disturbs that control, such as infection, injury or degeneration, that we become once more unable to control the muscle: this is known as being incontinent.

Incontinence in children
The child who has gained control over his bladder may become incontinent because of some interruption in the normal pattern of development. There may be a physical cause or an emotional one. Parents usually find it very distressing and clinics exist to help the family to overcome the problem.

Another worry is the child who is exceptionally late in gaining control over his bladder. Many children develop slowly and parents often forget how difficult it is for a child to accept enforced delay, even after he has gained control of his bladder. Staying dry at night is often seemingly impossible to achieve, but parents should not give up hope of their child ultimately achieving full control over his bladder until he is at least eight years old.

Stress incontinence
Many women suffer from stress incontinence, especially after childbirth. This means that whenever anything like sneezing, coughing or laughing raises the intra-abdominal pressure, urine escapes involuntarily, causing a considerable degree of embarrassment and discomfort.

The condition is due to the stretching of the ligaments and muscles that support the womb (uterus). The womb drops and in so doing presses on the bladder. This is known as a prolapse. If discomfort is severe or prolonged, the condition can be cured by an operation.

Incontinence in older men
The older man may sometimes find it difficult to pass urine even though his bladder is full (a condition known as retention of urine). This is because the prostate gland, which encircles the top of the urethra (see page 80) has become enlarged and is making it difficult for urine to get past. The bladder becomes overfull and eventually urine dribbles out (retention with overflow). Like stress incontinence, this type of incontinence can also be successfully treated by an operation.

Incontinence in the physically handicapped
Anyone who has damage to the spinal cord and who is a paraplegic has lost control of his bladder. Emptying of the bladder is therefore involuntary and intermittent. Some of these patients are eventually able to relearn control, but some may have to rely on incontinence aids permanently (see pages 86-87).

Incontinence in the elderly

By far the largest group of sufferers from incontinence are the elderly. They may lose control of the bladder or their decreased mobility may simply make it impossible for them to reach the lavatory in time.

The inability to wait: Urgency may be the result of infection, which the doctor may treat with antibiotics. The problem may also be one of mobility. Old people need to get to the lavatory quickly when their bladders are full. If their movements are too slow accidents occur. Some old people have arthritic hands and find adjusting their clothing difficult. This problem should be considered when new clothes are bought and velcro could be used to replace fastenings on existing garments (see page 54). Regular visits to the lavatory (especially after meals), walking aids, and, if possible, a room near the lavatory will all help.

Patients with speech difficulties may be unable to ask for a bedpan.

True incontinence: This means that all bladder control is lost. The brain no longer controls the function and the bladder acts as it does in the baby: it empties suddenly, frequently and involuntarily. The loss of control may be only temporary, depending on the extent of the brain damage: after a minor stroke, for instance, control is eventually regained; but after severe damage, loss of control is permanent.

Helping the Incontinent Patient

A great deal can be done to help the incontinent patient who, already humiliated and distressed, must not also be made to feel a nuisance. The bladder tends to respond to a routine, so a regular visit to the lavatory every two to three hours may help. An alarm clock or kitchen "pinger" can be used as a reminder. Patients should be encouraged to drink, for cutting down on fluids makes the condition worse, not better. However, it is sensible to control fluid intake late in the day.

It is important to avoid constipation: include fresh fruit, vegetables and roughage in the patient's diet every day.

When urine is passed involuntarily, attend to the patient promptly. Wash and dry the skin thoroughly but gently, and apply a waterproof cream. If the patient is up and about, special pants with disposable liners can be used, but these may not be a satisfactory full-time solution as plastic causes sweating, which can lead to soreness. During the night, absorbent drawsheets and pads may be advisable. A urinal or commode can be left near the bed for the patient's use.

Supplementary benefits are available for extra expenses associated with incontinence, such as laundry, heating, bedding replacement, floor coverings or special clothing. Many areas run a laundry service for the incontinent patient, washing and drying (but not ironing) bedlinen, nightclothes and underclothes. Collection and delivery are arranged on a regular basis.

Where incontinence cannot be treated, personal protection is essential. To feel dry and confident of being odour-free is a morale-booster. There is much help available that is never used. Suitable clothing is described on page 54, while machine washable shoes or plastic shoes that can be scrubbed help to prevent odour. Advice and many aids can be obtained through the family practitioner and district nursing sister (see page 86-87). Unfortunately many patients and relatives are too embarrassed to seek advice. They tend to isolate themselves as the laundry piles grow higher.

As a volunteer you can do much to make people aware of the help available. You may also be in a position to help and encourage the relatives, who often feel incontinence is a problem to be tackled only by professionals and are therefore reluctant to admit any responsibility themselves for supporting the patient.

Aids for the Incontinent

Any aids recommended should be chosen with the individual needs of the patient in mind. These will vary depending on whether the patient is incontinent only at night or in the daytime too, and on whether he is up and dressed or in bed for most of the day. The age and condition — physical and mental — of the patient should also be taken into account.

Urinals for men are especially valuable at night when the patient cannot be moved. Female urinals are small and light. They hold 600ml and can be slipped between a patient's legs without her hips needing to be raised off the bed. A Feminal consists of a plastic holder and a polythene bag. Specially moulded to the female shape, it can be used sitting or standing and is small enough to be carried in a handbag. If the bag cannot be emptied immediately after use and a new bag attached, it can be tied and kept for a while.

There are many types of incontinence pants suitable for men and women. Fitted pants are made of a soft material with a waterproof pouch on the outside. The urine passes straight through the pants to be absorbed by a pad placed in the pouch, so leaving the skin dry. The pants are worn with the pouch opening in front. To insert the pad double it over your hand and slide it into the pouch. This is made easier if the patient's knees are apart and the pants pulled down a little. Place the pad well in front for male patients and nearer the back for women. Change the pads as required and the pants daily. The pants may be hand or machine washed but should not be bleached. They are not suitable for being worn at night.

Stretch pants are light, open-stretch pants designed to fit any patient, whatever size. Across the pants are two woven-in blue bands which hold a plastic-backed

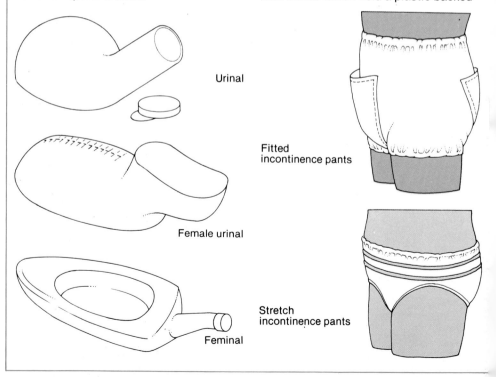

Urinal

Female urinal

Feminal

Fitted
incontinence pants

Stretch
incontinence pants

pad firmly in place. These pants can be used at night and can also be either hand or machine washed but not bleached.

Underpads are made of layers of absorbent material backed by waterproof material. There are various kinds. Pads are especially useful at night.

A Kylie bed sheet combines a drawsheet with an underpad. The central part is a soft absorbent yellow quilted material while the edges are thinner sheeting for tucking in. The centre allows urine to spread across it.

The sheet may be left under the patient for 12 hours. It never feels really wet, just damp when saturated. It looks and feels pleasant and can be frequently laundered. A spin dryer is needed as their absorbency makes these sheets extremely heavy. Unfortunately, they are expensive and you would need at least two.

The use of pants and pads as incontinence aids should not mean that regular visits to the lavatory are abandoned.

When disposing of soiled pads or pant liners first place them on newspaper, never on an unprotected floor. Wrap them up and place them in a plastic bag. The plastic bags for the disposal of incontinent or surgical waste may be provided through the local district authority or local health authority. The district nursing sister will advise you how to get hold of them.

To give the patient more independence a catheter may be inserted into the bladder and left in position. This is known as long-term catheterization. The urine drains into a bag strapped to the leg or supported by a waist belt. The bag is emptied periodically. The problem is that catheters encourage infection. They must be changed regularly by a doctor or nurse and the area around them must be kept clean. Follow the advice of the district nursing sister: she may suggest washing carefully around the catheter with soap and water, using a flannel kept for this purpose only. Alternatively the patient may be given a daily bath if he is fit enough.

Some male patients are fitted with rubber sheaths (condoms) attached to tubing which drains into a bag attached to the leg.

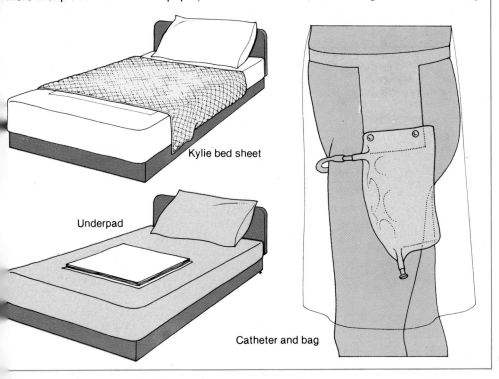

Kylie bed sheet

Underpad

Catheter and bag

Faecal Incontinence

Inability to control the bowel is a rarer problem than losing control of the bladder. It may be caused by a bowel infection or, occasionally, by a severe psychological disturbance (most common in childhood). Another cause is severe constipation, when an accumulation of faeces partly blocks the intestinal passage. If it is so severe that the faeces begin to decompose and become fluid, frequent and involuntary bowel movements occur as the more liquid faeces seep past the obstruction and leak out. The condition can be treated with diet and fluids.

The Patient with a Stoma

In the treatment of certain diseases of the digestive tract, it may become necessary to remove part of the tract. Whenever possible the two cut ends of the tract are sewn together to maintain a passageway for food and waste materials. When this is not possible, an artificial opening (or stoma) is made in the abdominal wall through which undigested material can pass into a bag.

People with colostomies may wear bags fixed permanently underneath their clothing. The bags can be of different types. They may be supported on a special belt or — as here — they may merely be attached to the skin around the stoma with adhesive.

Colostomy

A colostomy is when the contents of the colon or large bowel are made to bypass the rectum and the colon is brought on to the surface of the stomach. The faeces then pass through an opening in the abdominal wall. They are fairly firm and their consistency can be controlled with diet and medicines. The patient may wear a bag and belt underneath his clothing, but once the stools are formed and regular, he may manage with just a dry dressing over the opening, exchanging this for a bag only when a bowel movement is expected. A well regulated colostomy acts once a day: the patient can deal with it as if it were a normal rectal opening and then forget about it.

Ileostomy

The ileostomy is when part of the small intestine, the ileum, is brought to the surface of the stomach. This is much higher up the gut than a colostomy and the faeces passed are much more fluid. The patient requires a bag permanently in position; it must be leak-proof, unobtrusive under clothing and easy to deal with.

Helping to Care for a Stoma

Anyone seeing a stoma for the first time may feel revolted by it. This includes the family, the volunteer and the patient. Everyone feels distaste for the abnormal, and the idea of faeces being discharged on to the abdominal wall is abnormal.

The patient is distressed because he lacks bowel control; he is anxious in case he gives offence through odour or by soiling his clothes and he is embarrassed in case his appliance shows through his clothing. Relatives and friends may not be quite sure how to treat the patient: should you ignore the condition or try and offer sympathy? A simple acceptance of the situation often helps the patient most. The volunteer should be sensitive to the patient's feelings and in no way show any distaste. You must be gentle and confident when helping the patient with the stoma and so make the patient feel that this is a routine procedure and no more unusual than giving a bedpan.

While the patient is still in hospital after the operation, a suitable appliance should be selected. The skin around the stoma will need special care to prevent it from becoming sore. The patient's diet may also need adjusting and disposal of used bags may seem to present a problem. Once it is controlled, the stoma should present no special problem as long as it is attended to once a day.

Your role is to ensure that the patient can deal with his stoma in privacy if he cannot go to the bathroom. He will need a bowl of warm water, soap and a towel to wash and dry the surrounding area. He should also have a paper bag in which to dispose of the full bag and a fresh one to take its place.

When the patient has finished, remove the tray and dispose of the faeces by cutting across the top of the bag and emptying its contents into the lavatory. A pair of scissors should be kept separate for this purpose; they should be washed and dried after use. The bag can be wrapped in newspaper, burned or placed in the dustbin. Give the patient a fresh bowl to wash his hands when he has finished.

Patients become very skilled at adjusting their own diets and protecting their skin from damage. If there are any problems consult the family doctor or district nursing sister. There are also specialist societies who can give the patient and his family help and support (see *Useful Addresses*).

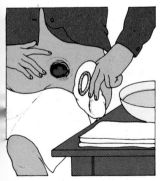

1 The patient removes the full colostomy bag and disposes of it into a paper bag placed ready nearby.

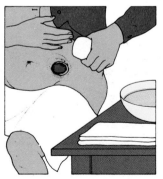

2 With warm water and soap she washes the stoma and the skin of the surrounding area.

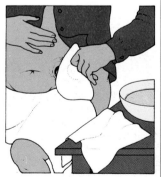

3 After she has dried the stoma with a towel, she has a new colostomy bag ready to put in position.

Changing the New Baby

Babies pass urine frequently and should never be left in a wet napkin. Some babies pass urine at regular times but most do not. Every time you change the napkin you should wash the buttocks with soap and water, or with baby lotion, if preferred. You should then dry them well and apply a protecting and soothing baby cream before putting on a clean napkin.

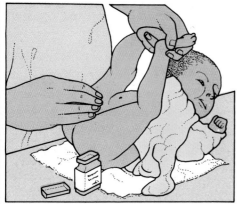

The easiest way of changing a young baby is to hold her ankles together with one hand and lift her buttocks off the changing surface.

Stools

Before a baby is born its gut is full of a dark green sticky material called meconium. This is passed within a few hours of birth and continues for about three days, after which time it becomes light brown in colour and is known as a changing stool. On about the fourth or fifth day the stool takes on a curdy bright yellow appearance. Breast-fed babies continue to pass soft stools, while bottle-fed babies pass stools which are more solid and formed, smell more like ordinary stools and are usually passed less frequently than those of the breast-fed baby. Once weaning commences, the stools change again, becoming still darker in colour and firmer in consistency.

Napkin rash

In certain circumstances the baby's buttocks may become red and sore. It is important to change napkins frequently, to wash and dry the baby's buttocks carefully, and to rinse out napkins adequately every time. Diarrhoea may also be a cause of sore buttocks. The application of a soothing cream, such as zinc and castor oil cream, helps to protect the skin with a waterproof layer while soothing the sore area. If none of these precautions seems to make any difference, you should seek the advice of your doctor.

Types of napkin

The main decision is whether to use washable napkins or disposable ones. There are advantages and disadvantages associated with both.

The basic washable napkin is usually a terry towelling square, quick-drying but highly absorbent when folded to the baby's shape. Gauze squares can be used for very new babies and as napkin liners later on.

Disposable napkins are absorbent pads with plastic backs. They are less absorbent than washable nappies, but they are certainly convenient if washing facilities are limited.

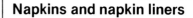

Napkins and napkin liners

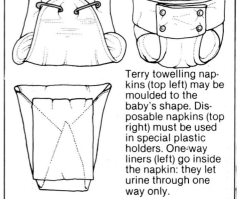

Terry towelling napkins (top left) may be moulded to the baby's shape. Disposable napkins (top right) must be used in special plastic holders. One-way liners (left) go inside the napkin: they let urine through one way only.

Types of plastic pants

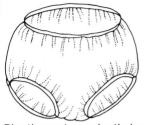
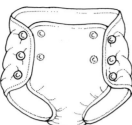
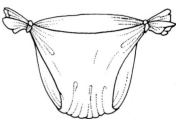

Plastic pants or plastic backing must be used with disposable napkins, and can be used with towelling napkins if desired. Although plastic pants are effective in keeping moisture off clothing and bedding, they tend to encourage redness and soreness. The best are probably the pants which tie like a napkin (top right). These offer some protection while still allowing air to circulate.

Sterilizing Napkins

Wet napkins must be properly washed and rinsed, so that ammonia from the urine or detergent from the wash does not come into prolonged contact with the baby's skin. Soiled napkins must be sterilized to avoid any danger of infection.

It is best to buy a special napkin sterilizing solution and two plastic buckets with lids. You should be able to tell the two buckets apart. Start by filling them both with napkin sterilizing solution. Drop wet napkins into one and soiled napkins into the other (first scraping off the worst of the soiled material into the lavatory). Do this every time you change a napkin in the course of the day. The solution needs changing every 24 hours and to be effectively sterilized napkins need at least six hours in the solution. This means that, assuming you start in the morning, any napkins you change during the night are best stored in a plastic bag and saved for the morning's new solution.

Every morning when you change the solution, rinse out the wet napkins. They do not need to be washed with detergent, but they must be rinsed thoroughly. The soiled napkins must be washed in very hot water with detergent before being thoroughly rinsed. Napkins stored during the night can go straight into the fresh solution.

This method of sterilizing napkins avoids constant washing and rinsing through the day, while also saving unnecessary washing.

Napkins should be dried outdoors if possible or in a tumble-dryer. If they are put to dry on radiators or hot pipes they will become unpleasantly stiff and abrasive when put next to the baby's skin.

Napkin sterilizing solution is very strong and contains bleach. This means that coloured garments must be washed separately, even if soiled. You should also avoid any prolonged contact with the solution. Most important is never to touch the baby's delicate skin before rinsing the solution off your hands.

Two large plastic buckets with lids can be used to hold sterilizing solution.

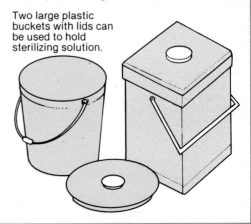

Methods of Putting On Napkins

There are many different ways of putting on napkins, depending on the sex and size of your baby. Remember never to leave safety pins open while you are changing a napkin. For added safety always secure pins horizontally rather than vertically.

The triangle method
Fold the napkin in half so that it forms a triangle. Fold down the edge, taking account of the baby's size. Lay the baby on the napkin with its apex between his legs. Bring the three corners together and fasten with one safety pin.

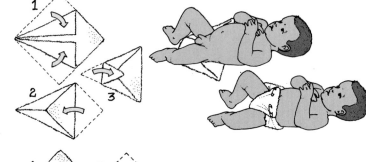

The kite method
Fold in the left and right hand corners until they meet. Fold down the top corner to make a triangle. Fold up the lower point. Lay the baby on the napkin. Bring the sides together and fasten them with two safety pins.

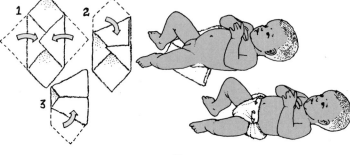

The parallel method
Fold the top and bottom corners of the napkin so that they overlap. Fold in the left corner until its top edge is level with the top fold. Fold in the right corner in the same way. Lay the baby on the napkin and fasten the sides with two safety pins.

The rectangle method
Fold the napkin in half. For a girl fold the top down one-third; for a boy fold the bottom up one-third. Lay the baby on the napkin. Bring the sides together and fasten them with two safety pins.

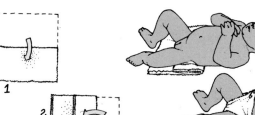

REST AND SLEEP:
Helping the patient to relax and maintain good sleeping habits

REST AND SLEEP

Everyone is familiar with the tiredness and listlessness that commonly follow a late night. Other symptoms are headache, little interest in food and, above all, little energy to face the new day. In these circumstances, your body is suffering from the lack of sleep imposed on it.

The healthy person who sleeps well wakes up feeling physically energetic and mentally refreshed. The sick person needs more rest than the healthy one to restore energy. This is because in sickness, the body must repair the damage caused by infection, injury or disease. For this it needs plenty of rest, so that it can build up the reserves of energy necessary to fight infection and illness.

As part of your nursing care, therefore, you must make sure that the patient is getting enough sleep, so that both body and mind are relaxed. At the same time, recognize the value of rest for its own sake. Rest is restorative: a patient who finds sleeping difficult will benefit from being encouraged to relax and rest even if he does not go to sleep. The chances are, however, that a relaxed and drowsy patient will eventually fall asleep.

Helping the Patient

To help a patient rest and sleep you need to know something about his normal sleeping pattern. If he is waking up every morning in the early hours, his need for help will obviously depend on whether he usually sleeps through the night or not. You need to find out if normally he goes to bed early or late and if he is used to a nap in the afternoon. Perhaps he sleeps a great deal during the day because he works at night; perhaps he is used to a hot drink or a tot of alcohol last thing at night.

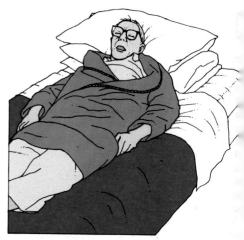

It is when a person's normal pattern is disturbed that he has the most difficulty in sleeping, so learn to be sensitive to it: if you bring him a cup of tea at the very moment when he usually takes half an hour's nap, the patient may find it harder, not easier, to get to sleep that night.

Causes of Wakefulness

There are many types of disturbance that can prevent a tired patient from relaxing into sleep. Some of these are practical and may prevent sleep on one isolated occasion: these should be relatively easy for you to assist the patient in resolving. Other problems may prevent him from getting enough sleep night after night, without there being any obvious or simple solution. In these cases, identification of the cause is still the first step to take, even if this does not necessarily mean that a permanent answer to the problem is any easier to find immediately.

Environment

Consider the patient's environment. Is he in his own bedroom? A change of surroundings can be very disturbing, and it is not only the patient in hospital who suffers but the patient at home who is being nursed in a different room for practical convenience. If unfamiliarity of surroundings is keeping the patient awake, all you can do is try and leave the rest of his routine as unchanged as possible.

The patient may not be happy with the temperature of his room at night, especially if he himself is feverish. Is the room well ventilated without draughts and are the bedclothes warm enough for the time of year without being too heavy? One blanket more or less may make a surprising difference to the patient's comfort.

Is the room free from smells? The sense of smell is heightened in illness. The patient may be nauseated by cooking smells, stale flower water too near the bed or bedpans not removed immediately after use. Remember to use an air freshener in the bedroom after he has had a bowel action. The patient may even be disturbed by the smell of his own body. Discharges from a wound or stale sweat (particularly if the patient has a limb in plaster) can be extremely distressing. Wash the skin often, using a deodorant where appropriate and leave a pleasant-smelling aerosol within the patient's reach so that he can use it whenever he wishes to do so.

The amount of light may disturb the patient's sleep. If his condition warrants a night nurse or night sitter, there must be a light so that she can see the patient but it should be carefully shaded to avoid disturbing him. Conversely, the child used to a small nightlight may be afraid of the darkness if he is left without one.

Discomfort

People normally differentiate between night and day by wearing different clothes. It may help an ill person to feel more normal if he can also change into clean pyjamas or a fresh nightdress to sleep. Wrinkled sheets, crumbs in the bed and untucked bedclothes all contribute to restlessness. Because of this, always see that the sheets are pulled taut and smooth when you are settling the patient to sleep and that he is comfortably settled on pillows. This is especially important if the patient is totally confined to bed. The lack of any change of scene and the consequent feelings of frustration and boredom serve to intensify even the slightest discomfort. Check also that the bedclothes are not too heavy, although some patients are used to weight and miss it if it is removed — if blankets are replaced by a continental quilt, for instance.

Make sure that a patient with breathing difficulties is comfortably supported with pillows. If something is irritating his skin or there is undue pressure on any part of it, this needs special attention (see page 29). A swollen limb may be more comfortable raised on a pillow, while painful joints are often eased if the bedclothes are supported by a bed-cradle.

A full bladder is a common cause of sleeplessness, especially if the patient is reluctant to call anyone during the night and cannot get out of bed. Always offer a bedpan or urinal when settling the patient for the night and allow plenty of time for him to use it. If he is fairly mobile, he may like to have a bedpan, urinal or commode beside him during the night.

Indigestion may be relieved with peppermint water or a simple indigestion tablet, while nausea can often be relieved with soda water. Coughing may be helped by a change of position, together with extra pillows and a spoonful of honey or lemon. If the particular discomfort that disturbs the patient *can* be alleviated by a simple remedy, reassurance will help to relax him and prepare him for sleep.

Hunger and Thirst

The sick patient is often reluctant to eat and yet he may well feel both hungry and thirsty during the night. Although a large fluid intake last thing at night is probably unwise, a milky drink taken last thing before settling to sleep is often the answer. Stimulants such as tea and coffee, however, are best avoided unless the patient usually drinks these late at night.

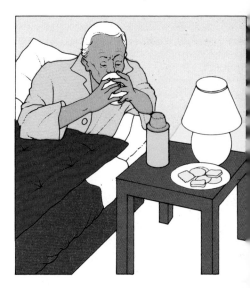

If the patient is feverish or the weather very hot, a jug of lemon squash or lemon barley water is refreshing. Many older people are used to a tot of alcohol at night: there is no harm in this unless expressly forbidden by the doctor.

If the patient wakes in the early hours of the morning feeling hungry or thirsty, a few biscuits or a hot drink left on his bedside table may soothe him to sleep again.

Noise

Noise disturbs sleep. Unfortunately, it is often those caring for the sick who make the most noise. For this reason, wear quiet shoes and clothing that does not rustle. Try and eliminate noises in cisterns and radiators if you can. Close doors quietly and make sure that they cannot swing open and shut in a sudden draught.

Absolute quiet can also be disturbing, especially during the day, so do not eradicate all the sounds of normal living. Simply keep the television, radio, record-player or sounds of playing children a little more subdued than usual.

Fears and Anxieties

Fear undoubtedly keeps people awake. The sick person always has fears, and it is pointless to pretend that they do not exist. In the hours of darkness they may loom especially large and seem most threatening. The patient may have many different worries: How long shall I get pay? Can we manage on sickness benefit? Shall I be fit to do my old job when I am better? Shall I get my old job back? Shall I be disfigured? Shall I still be attractive to my boyfriend or husband? Am I becoming a burden as I get older? Who will look after me when I cannot cope any longer? Shall I be able to bear the pain? Am I going to die?

All these are very real anxieties, some without solution. Yet there is truth in the old adage that a burden shared is a burden halved. Try and get the patient to *talk* to you: give him your full attention and listen properly. Most of the time you are probably so busy that even when the patient is talking to you, you do not *really* listen. On the other hand, be careful not to pry. At night, when the patient is in low spirits he may find it possible to talk to a sympathetic listener, but the next day he may wish he had not confided in you and may not want to be reminded of your conversation the night before.

Pain

Perhaps the greatest enemy of sleep is pain. Pain can be increased by any or all of the factors discussed above, while attention to these factors will minimize and perhaps even remove the pain.

The doctor should always be told about any persistent pain. He will want to know what the pain is like, when it usually occurs and whether anything in particular seems to cause it.

Pain-killing drugs and sleeping tablets may be prescribed by the doctor, but should only be given in accordance with his instructions.

The New Baby

A newborn baby has not yet established a sleeping pattern. He will sleep when he needs to sleep for as long as his body tells him to do so. Most babies sleep for between 16 and 20 hours a day in the first few weeks of life, but some may sleep for less time from the very beginning. He will sleep progressively less as he grows: by the time he has reached the age of five the average child is sleeping about 12 hours a day.

The newborn tends to wake when he is hungry or uncomfortable. He does not distinguish night from day and wakes at random through the 24 hours. It takes several weeks before the baby starts to be awake during the day more than at night. He will adjust sooner if he is put down to sleep in different places: at night, for instance, he may sleep in his cot while during the day he may be in his pram in a room with the window open and with older brothers and sisters playing round him. Their noise will not keep him awake if he needs to sleep.

In fine weather the baby can sleep outside, in a sheltered spot where the sun will not shine directly on to the pram. Protect the pram with a cat net and make sure the brake is on.

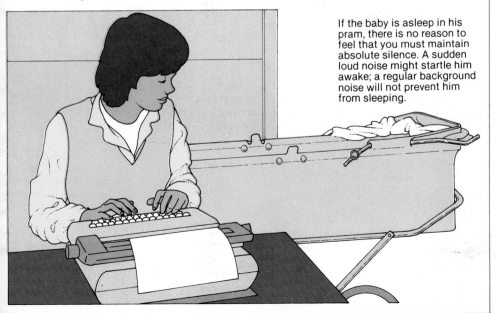

If the baby is asleep in his pram, there is no reason to feel that you must maintain absolute silence. A sudden loud noise might startle him awake; a regular background noise will not prevent him from sleeping.

The Sick Child

When a child is feeling really ill he will lie still in bed. He will doze or sleep as much as his body dictates until he starts to feel better. All you need to do is to keep him comfortable in pleasant surroundings and give him plenty of love and attention when he is awake.

At the next stage of illness, in early convalescence, you may need to take more active steps to make sure that the ill child is getting enough rest and sleep. The child is feeling better and will therefore be more active and restless. He will be easily bored and inclined to be mischievous. He will move about as much as he can and easily become overtired, while at the same time finding it harder to rest.

It is important that at this stage you provide lots of entertainment to keep the child's mind occupied and his body rested: jigsaws, stories and as much attention as possible. If the child is busy but physically relaxed, he will sleep better at night. Even a relaxed child, however, may be kept awake by fear and anxieties, which may or may not be related to his illness.

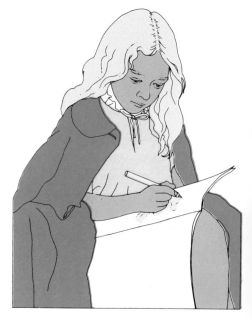

Night Fears

Night fears are common in childhood anyway but they may be accentuated by illness. The sick child probably needs more comforting than usual and may have many apparently irrational fears — of the bogey man coming to take him away or of some other fantasy person in the room. Do not dismiss his fears too easily. Instead put your head down to his level and look at the room from his angle: you may get a surprise. Nightlights can cast dramatic shadows which look extremely threatening. Moving the light will usually remove both the shadow and the fear. However, like the adult, the child may have fears associated with his illness. Reassurance and understanding together with a cuddle are probably the most soothing way of helping him to sleep.

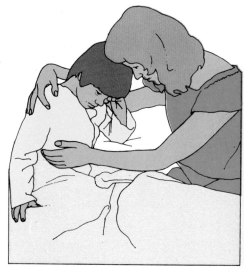

CONTROLLING TEMPERATURE: Helping the patient to maintain normal body temperature

CONTROLLING TEMPERATURE

In spite of wide variations in environmental temperature, man's body temperature stays remarkably constant. Its normal range is between 36° and 37°C. The healthy body achieves a balance between the heat it produces and the heat it loses. The amount of heat lost from the skin is modified by the type of food eaten and the clothing worn.

Extreme heat is usually counterbalanced by the heat regulating mechanism in the brain, which cools the body down by causing increased sweating. When the balance between heat loss and heat gain is disturbed, it is a sign that the patient has got some kind of infection (or injury). When only parts of the body are affected certain local reactions occur: this is known as inflammation. Where the whole body is involved in overcoming infection, the body temperature rises: if it goes above 37°C this is known as fever or pyrexia. If extreme cold causes the body to lose more heat than it can produce, body temperature may fall as low as 32°C: this is hypothermia.

Hypothermia

The basic cause of hypothermia is a lack of external heat combined with the body's inability to produce sufficient insulation. The heat loss from the body is greater than the heat produced and the body temperature falls abnormally low. The loss of surface heat is followed by cooling of the deep tissues and organs of the body.

Young, fit adults exposed to extremely low temperatures can die from hypothermia if they are inadequately clothed, sheltered and fed. Each year several climbers and walkers die from exposure. In the home, however, it is young babies and the elderly who are at risk, especially during the winter months. If hypothermia is suspected, a special low reading thermometer (30° - 38°C) must be used.

Dealing with a Low Temperature

The newborn baby

The heat regulating mechanism in the brain of a newborn baby is not yet working efficiently so that he relies on his surroundings to maintain his temperature. It is therefore essential to make sure that a baby is kept in a warm room, possibly with additional heat at night. If the baby's room seems cold when you enter it and there is no evidence of extra heating, take a look at the baby. A chilled baby will probably have red cheeks and look healthy. This is deceptive. His hands and feet may be red and swollen and feel cold to the touch. His movements will be reduced and he will be too lethargic to suck.

If you come across a baby in this condition, warm him gradually against your skin, perhaps by taking him into bed with you, while you wait for medical help to arrive.

When you take a young baby out of doors in cold weather, warm his pram with a hot water bottle either under the mattress or at the foot of the pram, with several thicknesses of blanket between the baby and the bottle. The baby himself should be warmly clothed and covered with several light but warm layers.

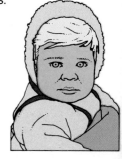

Unless the weather is very hot, a baby outdoors in her pram should have her head covered. Large amounts of heat are lost from the head, which in a baby is a particularly large proportion of the body.

The elderly patient

If when you arrive an elderly person is pale and his skin is cold to the touch, even where covered by clothing, suspect hypothermia. He may also be rather unsteady with slurred speech, slower and more confused than usual. His pulse may be slow and weak and his breathing slow and shallow. If you have a low-reading thermometer take his temperature. Send immediately for the doctor. In the meantime, wrap him in blankets and give him a hot drink to prevent him losing more heat. Do *not* use hot water bottles or electric blankets unless instructed to by the doctor. If you do, the sudden heat may make the surface blood vessels dilate and draw blood away from the deep tissues and vital organs, leading to a fatal collapse caused by a sudden fall in blood pressure.

Many elderly people say they do not feel cold when in reality they cannot afford adequate heating. If this is the case, you should persuade the person to get help from the Social Security Department. At the same time encourage the wearing of shawls, cardigans, mittens, bedsocks and — if the hair is thinning — for both sexes some kind of hat. It is surprising how much heat is lost from a bald head. Exercise will help blood circulate and tone up the muscles, even if it only consists of walking with you several times around the room. As room temperatures fall during the night, try and provide some kind of extra heating if possible: the ideal temperature is around 18°C. If there is a financial need, you can suggest that the elderly person uses one room only for living and sleeping, rather than heating two rooms or leaving a heated living room for a cold bedroom at night.

The elderly person should also be encouraged to eat a well-balanced diet; if necessary Meals on Wheels can be arranged, thus ensuring a hot meal at regular intervals (see page 64). Persuade him to take hot drinks during the day; perhaps you can leave a vacuum flask of hot fluid ready within his reach so that even if he is not very mobile he can drink frequently.

If an elderly person falls at night and is unable to summon help, his temperature may drop dangerously low. Where possible make sure that someone checks each morning to see that he is all right.

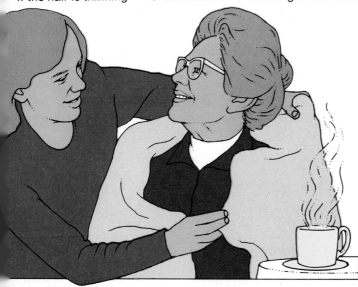

If you suspect that an elderly person is chilled when you visit her, take immediate measures to restore normal body heat. You can then go on to discuss what long-term measures might be taken to prevent the problem recurring. Of course, if you come across a patient who is severely chilled, you should seek medical advice at once.

Aids to Warmth

Electric blankets and bedwarmers

There are two types of electric blanket: one goes on top of the mattress under the patient and the other covers the patient. The underblanket should never be on when the patient is in bed, while the overblanket is safe enough to be left on when covering the patient, because it is attached to a transformer which reduces the voltage to 20 volts. Always follow the maker's instructions, and make sure that all blankets are in good condition, serviced regularly, and never allowed to get wet.

Bedwarmers are also electrically heated. They are metal containers, useful for warming a bed while the patient is up for a while. They heat a large area, especially if stood on one edge. Never leave one in bed with the patient.

This electric underblanket goes between the bottom sheet and the mattress.

An electric overblanket covers the patient.

Hot water bottles

Stone and metal bottles should only be used as bedwarmers and never when a patient is in the bed. More usual now are rubber bottles, which should be completely enclosed in a thick cover before being placed in the bed, on top of the first blanket. (Beware of bottles with a built-in cover: an exposed stopper may burn the patient.) Never use hot water bottles or heating pads in the beds of unconscious or paralysed patients, as the normal reaction to heat is lost and burning is likely.

Filling a hot water bottle

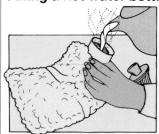

1 Lay a hot water bottle flat on a surface and fill it two-thirds full of water just off the boil.

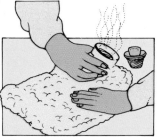

2 Expel the air by pressing against the surface before screwing in the stopper.

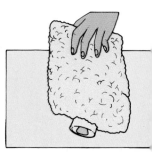

3 Wipe the top and invert the bottle to make sure it is not leaking before putting it in the bed.

Fever

You should know how to tell when a patient has a raised temperature (fever). You should also know what measures to take if it is not normal. It is important to keep the temperature under control to promote recovery. If your general impression is that the patient is feverish, you can confirm this by taking the patient's temperature (see page 104). As a routine procedure, however, this is not valuable. Indeed, over the years, much unnecessary time has been spent in taking and recording the temperature, pulse and respiratory rate.

The feverish patient is hot, bright-eyed, flushed and probably sweating. He may complain of a headache, feel thirsty, have a dry mouth and foul breath. In caring for him your priorities are:

- to make him feel cooler
- to quench his thirst
- to clean his mouth
- to deal with his headache.

Dealing with a High Temperature

There are several ways to make the patient cooler and more comfortable. A wash or blanket bath (see page 43) with a change of nightclothes and bedlinen is refreshing. You can remove some blankets and give the patient a bed cradle under his coverings so that air circulates. You can put an electric fan near the bed to move the air, as long as you do not chill the patient.

The feverish patient feels thirsty because he is sweating more than usual: sweat evaporates and cools the skin. Iced drinks are welcomed, especially sharp-flavoured ones. Frequent mouthwashes will moisten the mouth and freshen the breath.

As another result of the increased fluid loss, the patient may pass smaller quantities than usual of dark urine. If the fever lasts for more than a day or two he may also become constipated, partly because of fluid loss and partly because he is not eating very much. But most fevers are of short duration and small, light meals are adequate. Milky foods coat the tongue, so follow them with a mouthwash.

If his headache is severe, shade the patient's eyes from direct light and encourage him to rest quietly. A cold compress may be soothing, perhaps with a few drops of eau-de-cologne added to the water.

Applying a cold compress

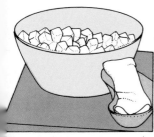

1 On a small tray put a bowl containing water and ice cubes. Fold a strip of linen or lint in three. Soak it in the iced water.

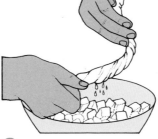

2 Wring the lint out by the ends of the strip to avoid warming up the centre.

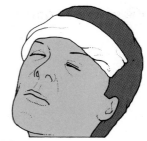

3 Apply the lint to the patient's forehead, and leave a second piece soaking in the bowl. Renew as necessary.

Factual Observations

To confirm your general impression of the patient's condition you may find it useful to take the patient's temperature, pulse and respiratory rate. Do not, however, write on the district nursing sister's home notes unless you are asked to. These are the notes she makes to record her nursing care, and they are used by the doctor to order treatment. She will usually leave the notes in an envelope in the same place after each visit, and you may look at them to see if there are any instructions for you. But if you have anything to report, write on a sheet of paper and slip it into the envelope. If, however, you are recording the temperature, pulse and respiratory rate, the doctor or nurse may ask you to use a temperature chart.

Taking the Temperature

In the mouth: This is the most usual method of temperature taking, suitable for most patients. But you should *not* take the temperature in the mouth if:
● the patient is unconscious
● the patient is a child or baby
● there is injury to the mouth such as a fractured jaw

● the patient is likely to have a fit
● the patient is confused.
  You use a clinical thermometer which should normally be stored in its case. If you are using it regularly, keep it dry in a small jar or in antiseptic. Before you take the temperature rinse the thermometer in cold water and dry it with a cotton wool swab.

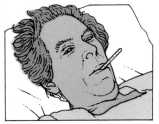 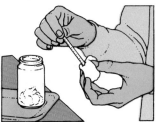 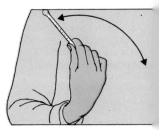

1 Shake the mercury down and place under the tongue. Ask the patient to close her lips, not her teeth.

2 Wait for two minutes. Remove, wipe the bulb, read and record the temperature.

3 Shake the mercury back down into the bulb and return the thermometer to the jar.

In the rectum: This method is used for babies and unconscious patients of any age. The rectal thermometer has a short bulb the same diameter as the stem. To take the temperature, you grease the bulb, gently insert it into the rectum and hold it firmly in position for two minutes. Then remove it, wipe, read and record the temperature. Shake down and replace in the antiseptic solution. When the temperature has been taken in the rectum this should be noted on the record. Rectal temperatures are a little higher than those recorded in the mouth.

In the armpit: The armpit (axilla) and groin may be used to record temperature if, for instance, the patient is subject to fits or if there is injury to the mouth. When the temperature has to be taken in the armpit, this should be noted on the record. Axillary temperatures are a little lower and less reliable than those recorded in the mouth. Both thermometer and skin must be dry. You lay the bulb in the armpit and fold the arm across the chest. After two minutes, remove it, wipe, read and record the temperature. Shake down and replace in the solution.

Disposable thermometers

Although not as accurate as conventional clinical thermometers, disposable thermometers are entirely safe and easy to use. They are especially suitable for babies and children.

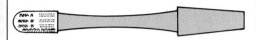

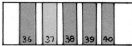

The thermometer is placed in the mouth for two minutes; the dot representing the temperature changes colour. The thermometer is then discarded.

A strip or disc is placed on the forehead for 15 seconds. The band recording the temperature changes colour. Both are re-usable.

Taking the Pulse

Each time the heart beats it pumps blood into the circulation, and a wave courses along the walls of the arteries. This wave is the pulse, which can be felt in the body at any point where a large artery crosses a bone just underneath the skin.

In a young baby the normal pulse rate goes up to 140 beats a minute, but during childhood the rate gradually falls. In the normal adult the rate is 60 to 80 beats a minute. There are many reasons for a rise in pulse rate: emotion, exercise, infection, shock, haemorrhage and heart disease are some of the most common. A fall in the pulse rate is more rare, but might be found in hypothermia.

As well as noting the rate, you should record the strength of the pulse — whether feeble, bounding or normal. Rhythm is also important: a normal pulse beats regularly.

It is important that you use your fingertips and not your thumb to take a pulse;

your thumb has its own pulse, and you risk counting that by mistake. It is essential to use a watch or a clock with a second hand for accurate counting. Practise on yourself and your friends until you feel confident.

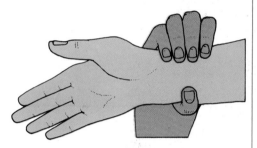

The easiest and most convenient place to feel the pulse is at the wrist, just above the crease on the thumb side. Sit the patient down. Place your fingertips over the pulse and support the patient's wrist with your thumb. Count the beats for one minute. Record.

Taking the Respiratory Rate

Each respiration consists of breathing in and breathing out, so the complete rise and fall of the chest is one respiration. The normal adult breathes 16 to 18 times a minute, but a higher rate is seen in many conditions: emotion, exercise, haemorrhage and diseases of the heart and lung are among the most common.

The rate at which a person breathes can be altered at will: anyone can breathe more quickly or slowly if he wants to. Once the

patient knows you are counting it becomes extremely difficult for him not to alter his respiratory rate. There is, therefore, no point in recording it unless you are trying to find out some definite piece of information, for instance about a respiratory infection.

To count the rate accurately, the patient must be unaware of what you are doing. The best time is when he is asleep; otherwise count the rate when you are at the bedside taking the pulse.

Inflammation

Inflammation is the body's response to injury or localized infection. The inflamed area may be small — a boil or a stye — or it may be extensive, with large quantities of pus forming an abscess. Whatever its size, it contains a large number of micro-organisms and precautions must be taken to prevent infection spreading from any open sore. These include:

● keeping the infected area covered
● placing soiled dressings in a paper bag straightaway and if possible burning them immediately
● otherwise wrapping the bag in newspaper and placing it in the dustbin.

It is most important for anyone who touches the wound or soiled dressing over an open sore to wash his or her hands thoroughly after attending to the patient, as otherwise there is a risk of micro-organisms being transferred from one person to another: this is known as cross-infection, but should not occur if proper precautions are taken.

Although infection is the major cause of inflammation, it is not the only one. After an injury such as a sprain the injured area is inflamed, and in diseases such as rheumatoid arthritis the affected joints are also inflamed. Inflammation also follows exposure to heat — burns and sunburn — or exposure to deep X-ray or radium. In all cases the signs are the same: the local irritation is dealt with by an influx of extra white blood cells and the increased blood supply makes the area red, hot and swollen. The patient complains of pain and is reluctant to use or move the affected part. Apart from these local signs, if the inflamed area is large the patient may have a raised temperature (see page 103).

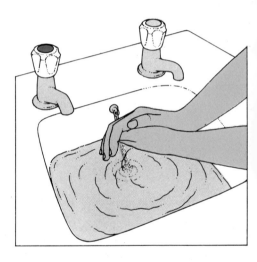

When you are dealing with a patient, especially if he has an open wound, it is absolutely vital to wash your hands thoroughly both before and after being in contact with him.

Caring for the Patient with an Inflammation

When caring for a patient with an inflammation, your priorities are:
● to reduce the swelling
● to relieve pain
● to remove the infection.

If the area is large, the patient should be in bed. If not, the inflamed area should be rested. If the inflammation is in a limb, the swelling and pain can be reduced by raising the part on a pillow: this encourages fluid to drain away. An arm can also be supported by a sling. The patient should drink at least three litres of fluid every day, to help remove impurities from the body. A mild pain-killer (an analgesic) may be prescribed and, if the infection is widespread, antibiotics may be ordered. In some cases a local application of heat may be effective.

Applying Local Heat

The application of heat to the affected area relieves pain and may localize the infection by increasing the blood supply to the area. Much of the treatment is often given by a physiotherapist in a specially equipped department. Radiant heat and short wave treatment are two methods of applying heat in common use.

In the home, warmed cotton wool or an electric pad can be laid against the area. A covered hot water bottle against the ear is most comforting if the patient has earache.

Making a kaolin poultice

Kaolin is a medicated clay, used to make a poultice. It is applied hot and renewed as ordered by the doctor.
You will need:
- a tin of kaolin
- a saucepan of boiling water

- a spatula
- a piece of old linen of appropriate size
- a piece of cotton wool about 2½ cm larger all round than the linen
- an ordinary bandage or an elasticized net bandage.

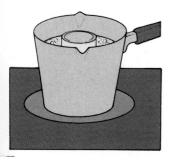

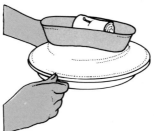

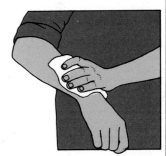

1 Place the tin of kaolin in the pan of boiling water with the lid of the tin on loosely; the water should not quite cover the top of the tin.

2 Spread the kaolin on to the linen when hot (making a poultice) and carry it to the patient between two warmed plates.

3 After testing the poultice on your forearm to make sure it is not too hot, apply it to the patient and cover with the cotton wool. Bandage in position.

Hot spoon bathing

This is a method of applying heat to the eye if the patient has a stye.
You will need:
- a wooden spoon
- cotton wool and gauze (or linen)
- a bowl of boiling water.

Pad the bowl of the spoon with wool. Cover it with a piece of gauze or linen and tie this securely around the handle. Sit the patient down and place the bowl of boiling water on a table in front of him. Let him put the spoon into the boiling water and then bring it up as close to his eye as the steam permits.

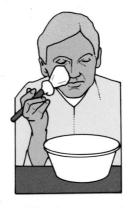

The patient should dip the spoon into the water and then bring it up as close to his eye as he can. As the water cools he will be able to bring it closer to the eye, so that it almost touches the lid. He should continue until the water is no longer hot.

Communicable Diseases

Fever is the outcome of a generalized infection and inflammation is the result of a localized infection. There is a special group of illnesses called the communicable or infectious diseases, all of which cause fever and the inflammation of the skin or glands. Serious communicable diseases are now relatively uncommon in Britain; those which do occur on the whole affect children more than adults.

All communicable diseases have certain characteristics:
- each illness is capable of being transmitted to others
- there is a specified time, known as the incubation period, between the infection of the body by the organism and the appearance of signs and symptoms
- in each illness every patient has the same signs and symptoms, although these may vary in the degree of severity
- most communicable diseases have a characteristic skin rash
- each disease lasts a certain number of days
- each disease is liable to cause complications, some of which are mild and some of which may be serious.

Modes of Infection

Communicable diseases are caused by micro-organisms: eaten with food or drink, breathed in from the air or entering through a break in the skin. They are spread by people and objects. They are carried by air and dust; by infected food, water and milk; by flies and rats; by infected bedlinen, crockery and books; by other people carrying the disease (carriers). Not everyone who is in contact with the micro-organism will contract the disease, because the body has defences against harmful organisms. It uses the white blood cells to destroy invading micro-organisms and the lymphatic glands to act as filters and remove them from the body for good.

A mobile baby will put to his mouth anything he comes across. Fluff on his toys may harm him; bacteria on old food certainly will.

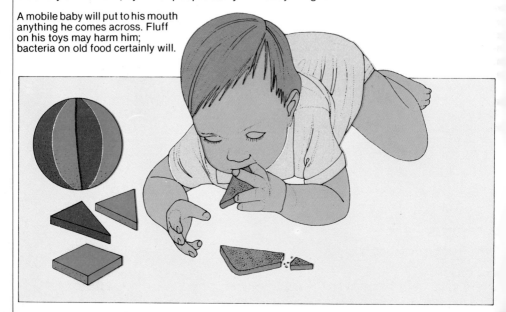

Caring for the Patient with a Communicable Disease

Your aim in caring for someone with a communicable disease is dual: to provide nursing care, and to prevent the spread of infection.

Nursing the patient

The type of care you will give the patient depends on the severity and seriousness of the illness. A child with a mild attack of German measles can be kept away from school for a few days and needs little nursing care. An adult with smallpox or poliomyelitis, on the other hand, will have to be admitted to a special isolation hospital and will require intensive medical and nursing care. In such hospitals, elaborate precautions are taken to protect the staff and to control the spread of infection.

As a volunteer you have no place in an isolation hospital, but you may well be involved in nursing an infectious patient in his own home. If this is the case, it is sensible for you to take certain precautions. Eat well and avoid becoming overtired. Wear an overall to protect your clothes and wash your hands carefully after attending to the patient. Turn away from him if he coughs or sneezes when you are attending to him. He should use paper handkerchiefs, which can be put in a paper bag and burned after use, or otherwise sealed in a plastic bag and put in the dustbin.

Keep visitors to a minimum and do not allow children near the patient unless the doctor says it is safe for them to visit. Some mothers keep their children together, in the hope that they will all have a disease at the same time. But this should be discouraged, as one child might develop serious complications.

The patient with a communicable disease will have a raised temperature and you should nurse him as you would any patient with a fever (see p. 103). If he also has an irritating rash, you can apply calamine lotion to cool and soothe the skin.

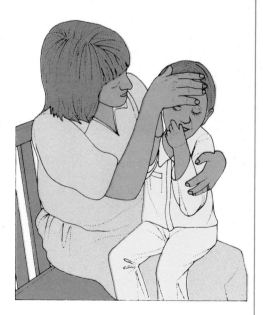

If a child is more clingy than usual and seems off-colour, just feeling his forehead will probably establish whether he is feverish.

Containing infection

There are several precautions you can take to help prevent the spread of infection. Nurse the patient in a well ventilated room where possible, with a window open except when he is being washed or treated.

Bedpans and urinals should be taken to the lavatory immediately after use and the contents flushed away. The district nursing sister will advise you if you need to take any other precautions.

INCUBATION AND ISOLATION PERIODS

Disease	Incubation period	Isolation of patient	Action to be taken for contacts	Availability of immunization
Chickenpox	11-21 days	Isolate for 7 days from onset of rash	None	No
Common cold	2-3 days	Whilst child is ill (2-5 days)	None	No
Conjunctivitis (purulent)	24-28 hours	Keep away from school until eye is clean	None	No
Diphtheria	2-5 days	Isolate until doctor advises	Medical Officer of Environmental Health (MOEH) will advise in every case	Yes
Gastro-enteritis (diarrhoea and vomiting)	Depends on cause	Isolate	Depends on cause	No
German measles (rubella)	14-21 days	Keep away from school for approximately one week	Children may continue at school but expectant mothers should not work at the school unless vaccinated	Available for girls aged 11-14
Impetigo	24-48 hours	While any scabs are exposed, the child should be away from school	None	No
Infective hepatitis	Varies — up to 3 months	Until doctor advises	None	Gamma globulin as preventive in special circumstances
Influenza	2-3 days	Keep away from school until recovered	None	Yes — in special circumstances
Measles (morbilli)	10-14 days	Keep away from school until doctor advises return.	None	Yes
Meningitis (several types)	Usually 2-10 days May be up to 2 weeks	Keep away from school until doctor pronounces fit	None	No

Disease	Incubation period	Isolation of patient	Action to be taken for contacts	Availability of immunization
Mumps (infective parotitis)	17-21 days	Keep away from school	None	No
Paratyphoid fever		See "Typhoid fever"		
Poliomyelitis	7-14 days	Keep from school until doctor pronounces fit	None	Yes
Ringworm of: body	Not known	No isolation required	Contacts will be seen by MOEH	No
feet	Not known	Some doctors advise the child should be excluded from swimming pools but this rule is not universally adopted	None	No
scalp	Not known	Keep away from school until doctor pronounces fit	Seen by MOEH	No
Scabies	Immediate on contact	Keep away from school until treated	MOEH will advise on home contacts	No
Scarlet fever		Same illness as tonsillitis, except that there is a rash		
Smallpox	8-17 days	Keep away from school until doctor pronounces fit	Contacts will be seen by MOEH	Though available not now given to all children
Tuberculosis	Usually 6 weeks	Keep away from school until doctor advises	Supervised by MOEH	BCG vaccination offers a degree of protection against certain forms of TB
Typhoid fever	Varies — usually about 2 weeks	Keep away from school until doctor advises	Contacts observed by MOEH	Sometimes given with paratyphoid vaccine and/or cholera.
Whooping cough (pertussis)	6-18 days	Isolate whilst child is infectious. Keep away from school until doctor advises.	None	Vaccination available for children under 3

Any food left on the patient's plate after he has finished should be removed and disposed of quickly.

Use a fly repellent spray to keep the bedroom and lavatory free of flies and insects.

Give the patient newspapers, magazines and paperback books to read that can be burned after use. If the patient has handled a library book, seal it in a plastic bag with sticky tape and return it to the librarian with an explanatory note. Try and give a child inexpensive toys that can either be burned or washed thoroughly after he has recovered from the illness.

You must be careful not to transmit infection yourself: wash your hands after attending to the patient, after emptying a bedpan, and whenever you leave the bedroom before handling anything else.

When the patient has recovered, strip the bed. Either send the linen to the laundry or wash it in a washing machine at a very hot setting. Open the windows and air the room thoroughly.

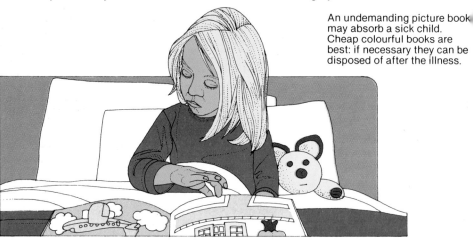

An undemanding picture book may absorb a sick child. Cheap colourful books are best: if necessary they can be disposed of after the illness.

Immunity

Once the body has been infected by a particular disease, it can produce antibodies which give life-long immunity to that disease — few people contract chickenpox, measles or mumps more than once. There is, however, no lasting immunity against some diseases — like the common cold — so the patient has repeated attacks.

Immunity can also be acquired by immunization. A worldwide immunization policy has resulted in the eradication of smallpox; in Britain immunization has almost eliminated diphtheria and poliomyelitis, and has greatly reduced the incidence of whooping cough, measles, tetanus and tuberculosis.

There is evidence that the number of children being immunized against these serious diseases is now falling. This may be partly the result of complacency born of ignorance — today's parents have not seen the effect of these diseases — and it may partly be fear that the vaccine used to immunize the child may be harmful. Recent publicity — about whooping cough for instance — has led to increased concern among parents. There is always a small risk in giving any vaccine, but the risk to young babies from whooping cough is generally considered far greater than the risk of the vaccine. If you are in doubt as to what you should do, talk to your doctor.

CARING FOR A WOUND: Helping the patient with an injury

CARING FOR A WOUND

A wound is a break in the skin, and may be the result of an injury or of an operation. Wounds need special treatment, depending on their size and severity. If they are severe enough, they may cause a raised temperature (see p. 103). Any adult can cope with cuts, grazes, and small burns or scalds; but, if the injury is larger, professional help may be needed and sometimes the patient may have to stay in bed or in hospital for many weeks.

However large or small the injury, the aim of nursing care is the same:
• to prevent bacteria entering the body and causing infection
• to hasten healing.

How a Wound Heals

When any part of the body has been destroyed by disease or injured in an accident, the adjacent tissues at once begin to repair the gap. This process is known as healing. A clean cut will heal more quickly than an area where tissue has been lost, such as a burn or an abscess.

When injury occurs, the wound bleeds and the space is filled with clotting blood. White blood cells begin to destroy and remove dead and damaged tissue. Cells grow rapidly into the clotted blood and form granulation tissue. Gradually this is replaced by firm, fibrous tissue. This is known as a scar. It is often red and a little raised, but eventually contracts and shrinks into a thin white line.

Healing is influenced by many factors. Tissues require oxygen and foodstuffs — especially vitamin C — in order to repair themselves. Age is important: babies and children heal much more rapidly than the elderly. If the general health is poor from a long illness or inadequate nutrition, the substances needed for healing will be in short supply. Vitamin C is then especially important. If the patient is anaemic he will require iron, so that the blood can carry sufficient oxygen for the tissues' needs. Finally, local irritants such as a foreign body or infection will also delay healing.

The patient should therefore be well nourished and have adequate vitamin C and iron in his diet. Rest is essential. Prevention of infection is also vital.

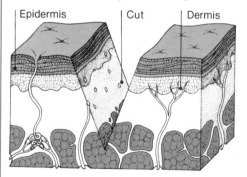

Epidermis | Cut | Dermis

Preventing Infection

The area must be cleaned so that any dirt is washed away and the wound must be covered with a dressing. A satisfactory dressing prevents bacteria from entering the wound but is porous enough to allow sweat to evaporate. If the dressing is not porous, the skin becomes moist, the dressing damp, and bacteria multiply.

The most efficient way of preventing infection from entering a wound is to eliminate bacteria from everything that comes into contact with the patient. This is done in two ways:
• by sterilizing equipment
• by using an aseptic technique when applying dressings.

Sterilizing Equipment

Bacteria are destroyed by fire, by steam under pressure, by boiling, gamma radiation or chemical disinfection. Once bacteria have been destroyed, the equipment can be used with safety. It is now usual for equipment to be sterilized either at the time of manufacture or in the Central Sterile Supply Department (CSSD) of a hospital.

Disposable equipment

Everyone is familiar with pre-packaged sterile dressings, which may be bought from the chemist. They are part of a range of items sterilized by the manufacturers. The equipment is sealed into plastic or paper covers and sterilized, often by exposure to gamma radiation from a nuclear reactor. Unless damaged, the equipment remains sterile until the seal is broken. For extra safety, many articles are wrapped in two covers.

Gauze dressings, cotton wool balls, paper towels, foil containers for lotions, instruments, syringes and catheters are in this way. Sometimes it is even possible to obtain small plastic sachets of sterile lotion.

For convenience, all the equipment and dressings needed to carry out a nursing procedure, perform a minor operation, or dress a wound, are often packed together and sealed in a paper bag or packet. This is sterile and ready for use at any time. After use, everything should be put into a paper bag, wrapped in newspaper and put in the dustbin or burned.

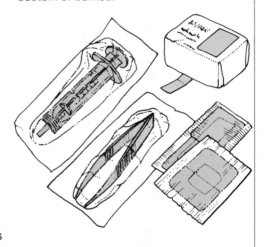

Non-disposable equipment

Some items (such as glass syringes, metal or polythene jugs and bowls) are too expensive to be thrown away after use. In hospital the Central Sterile Supply Department packs and sterilizes these items and delivers them to the wards and departments. After use, they are packed immediately in a paper bag, sealed and returned to the department where they are cleaned, repacked and sterilized ready for use once more.

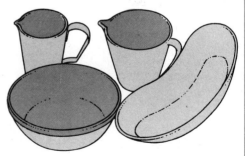

Checking before use

Inspect all sterile packages before use. If dated, check that the date has not passed. Check plastic packages to make sure they are not torn; check paper packages for wetness or for any staining that might suggest that they have been damaged by water at any stage.

Any package that allows fluid to penetrate, is torn or out of date, is no longer sterile and *must not be used*.

In an emergency most equipment can be adequately sterilized by immersing it in boiling water and boiling it for not less than three minutes.

Using an Aseptic Technique

In modern hospitals, a room is set aside for treatment but in older hospitals and in the home this is not possible. However, certain precautions should always be taken whenever a wound is dressed, to avoid contamination by micro-organisms. Avoid disturbing the air, as if dust and micro-organisms are moved, they may settle on the wound. For the same reason, avoid draughts and excessive movement. If the room needs cleaning, use a vacuum cleaner if possible or else sweep and dust the room at least one hour before applying a dressing, to allow the air time to settle. Clean any trays or trolleys to be used with soap and water and check that the sterile packets are undamaged.

Avoid unnecessary talking throughout the procedure, to keep the number of micro-organisms breathed out from the nose and mouth to a minimum. Wash your hands before you start.

What method you use to apply a dressing and how you secure it to the skin will depend on the size and position of the wound and on what equipment is available for you to use.

In the home, you are likely to be attending to a small graze, cut or burn, in which case the minimum of equipment is necessary. Occasionally you may assist the doctor or district nurse with a larger dressing but in these circumstances they will provide the necessary sterile equipment. Volunteers who are helping in the Accident and Emergency Department of a hospital or in a hospital ward will have sterile packs provided, which someone will show you how to use.

There are two methods of applying a dressing: one is just a clean method, while the other involves a 'non-touch' technique. There are several ways of securing the dressing, depending on the size and position of the wound (see p. 121).

Treating a small graze

The vast majority of dressings done in the home are to cover small grazes. The people most likely to suffer such grazes are children.

To dress a small graze, seat the patient and wash your hands thoroughly. Grazes often have dirt and grit embedded in them, so wash the area gently with soap and water until it is really clean. Then apply a self-adhesive dressing. Most dressings of this sort come off of their own accord a few days later. If you want to remove it, pull it off quickly rather than picking at it. The bath is a good place to remove old plasters. If you notice any redness around the dressing, take it off and examine the graze, for redness is a sign of infection.

Grazes are more painful than deeper wounds, because they expose an area of raw, tender skin full of sensitive nerve endings. A child who has grazed his skin needs a cuddle, plenty of attention and perhaps a sweet for bravery.

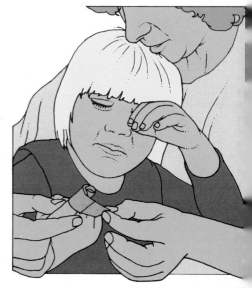

Even if a graze does not merit a plaster, a child will feel comforted if you put one on while you tell her how brave she is.

Treating a larger wound

For a larger wound, you will need:
- a tray
- cotton wool swabs and mild antiseptic
- a paper towel or square of kitchen roll
- the appropriate dressing
- a bandage or adhesive plaster
- a paper bag for soiled dressings
- a pair of scissors.

Seat the patient and expose the wounded area, removing any bandage or plaster already in place. Wash your hands thoroughly and gently clean the wound.

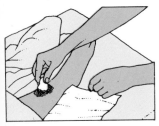 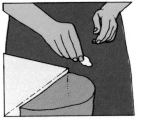 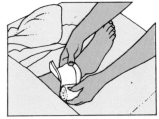

1 Hold the back of a cotton wool swab and wipe from the centre of the wound outwards.

2 Use each swab once only, discarding it immediately after use into the paper bag.

3 Cover the area with a clean dressing and secure it in position with a bandage or plaster.

Using a "non-touch" technique

This is a technique which might be used by the district nursing sister, in which case you might be asked to help her. It involves not touching anything that comes into contact with the patient and handling everything with forceps.

You will need:
- a tray or dressing trolley
- a sterile bowl for lotion
- sterile cotton wool swabs
- two sterile paper towels
- sterile gauze and wool dressings
- three or four pairs of sterile dressing forceps
- antiseptic lotion
- plaster removing solution
- a bandage or adhesive plaster
- a paper bag for soiled dressings
- a receiver for soiled instruments (if they are not disposable)
- a pair of scissors.

To apply the dressing, you proceed exactly as if you were applying an ordinary clean dressing, except that everything you use is sterile and is handled only with sterile forceps. You use two pairs of forceps

to remove the soiled dressing and two to clean the wound and apply the new dressing. When you have finished, everything is discarded into a paper bag and burned.

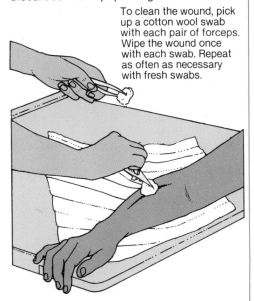

To clean the wound, pick up a cotton wool swab with each pair of forceps. Wipe the wound once with each swab. Repeat as often as necessary with fresh swabs.

Securing a Dressing

It is essential for dressings to remain in place, so they must be carefully secured. The way you secure a particular dressing depends on what type of dressing it is.

Adhesive dressings These are small pads of gauze with a waterproof adhesive backing, which is often perforated to let moisture evaporate. They are supplied in paper or plastic containers.

Prepared sterile dressings These are gauze pads covered by plain absorbent gauze and stitched to a roller bandage. They come wrapped in an outer cover and sterilized, and are useful dressings if nothing more specialized is at hand.

Adhesive plasters Strips of adhesive plaster can be cut from a roll to secure small dressings. Waterproof plasters are especially useful for areas such as the hands that are frequently exposed to water.

Stretch plasters These are used to cover quite large dressings. They also give some measure of support.

Clear adhesive tapes These are often used to hold small dressings in place, especially in areas where the skin is sensitive and might react to plaster, for instance around the eyes.

Plastic skin This can be sprayed on to a wound from an aerosol can. Many patients discharged from hospital have this type of dressing, which gradually flakes off.

Tubular gauze Especially useful for fingers and hands, tubular gauze makes a neat, firm bandage. It is supplied as a seamless roll, in various sizes to fit different parts of the body. You apply it with a special applicator. Apart from the finger size it is not

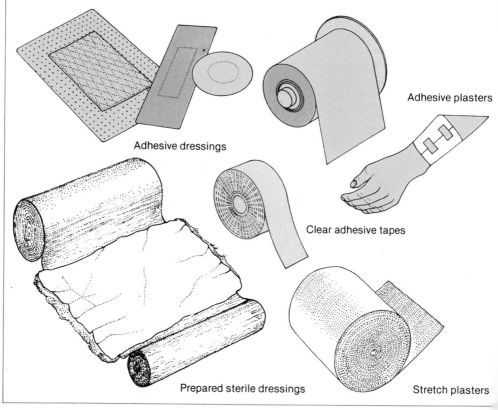

Adhesive dressings

Adhesive plasters

Clear adhesive tapes

Prepared sterile dressings

Stretch plasters

practical in the home, because it is expensive and you need a different applicator for each part of the body. If thought advisable for a patient at home, the district nursing sister would supply you with the appropriate applicator.

Elasticized net bandages Made of two-way stretch tubular mesh material, these bandages are easy to apply and comfortable to wear. They are especially valuable for securing dressings to difficult places such as the head, shoulder, thigh and groin. You cut the required length and stretch it over the dressing, cutting holes where appropriate to fit over limbs. These bandages do not fray when cut. You need a little practice to make sure of a good fit.

Roller bandages At one time, these were used extensively to keep dressings in posi-

tion, because they provided support while restricting movement. Nowadays, different methods are used for these purposes and roller bandages are applied less frequently. However, it is still useful to know how to apply a roller bandage.

Roller bandages are strips of material: they can be cotton, crepe, flannel, calico or special paper. They are five to six metres in length, and their width varies depending on the part to be bandaged and the age and size of the patient.

You will need:
- a width of 2.5cm to bandage a finger
- 5cm for a hand
- 5cm for a head
- 5 to 6cm for an arm
- 7.5 to 9cm for a leg
- 10 to 15cm for a trunk.

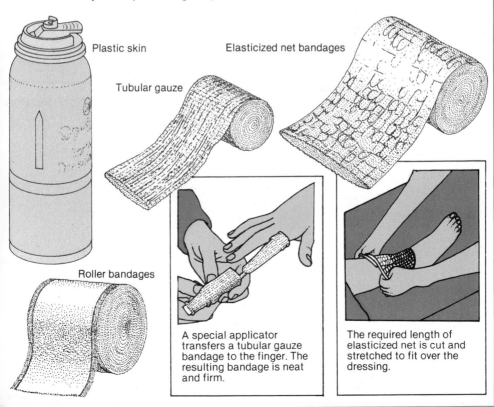

Plastic skin

Elasticized net bandages

Tubular gauze

Roller bandages

A special applicator transfers a tubular gauze bandage to the finger. The resulting bandage is neat and firm.

The required length of elasticized net is cut and stretched to fit over the dressing.

Applying a Bandage

Seat the patient comfortably and support the injured part. Always stand in front of the patient. Apply the bandage evenly and firmly. Too tight a bandage will restrict the patient's circulation and too loose a one will fall off.

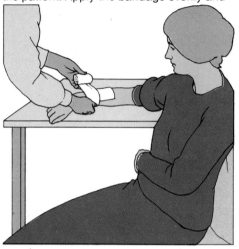

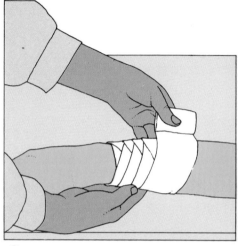

1 Hold the bandage with the roll uppermost and start to fix it around the wound with a firm turn.

2 Apply it from inside outwards and from below upwards. Use a firm even pressure for every turn.

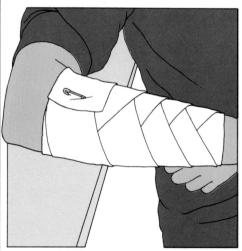

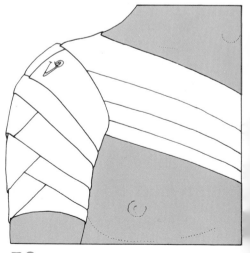

3 With each turn cover two-thirds of the previous one. Avoid covering the tips of fingers and toes. Fasten off the bandage with a small safety pin or bandage clip.

If two skin surfaces could rub and become sore under the bandage, for instance under the armpit, pad the part with cotton wool to avoid friction.

Bandaging Patterns

Simple spiral

This pattern can only be used when the part to be bandaged is of uniform size — for instance, a finger or forearm. The bandage is applied in straight turns around the limb.

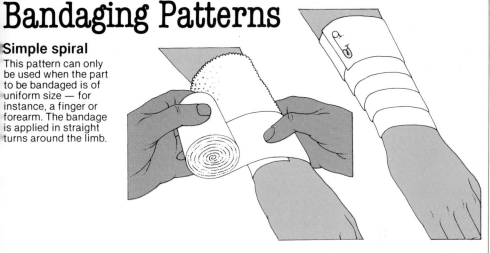

Figure of eight

This pattern is used for bandaging the arm or the leg. The bandage starts below the wound and progresses up the limb by encircling it in an '8' pattern.

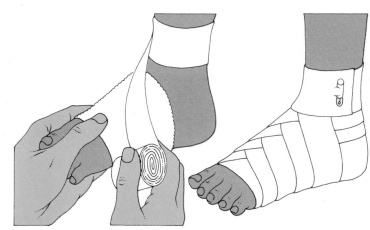

Divergent spica

This pattern is a variation on the figure of eight used for a flexed joint, such as a knee or elbow. Figure of eight turns are applied to the limb below and above the joint.

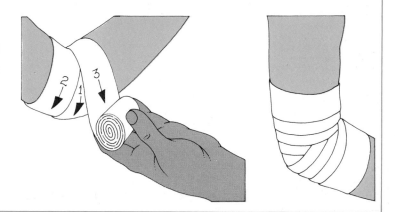

Making a Triangular Bandage

Any wound will heal better if it is rested. A lower limb should be rested on a stool or bed; an upper limb can be rested on a pillow or put in a sling. When you need to make a sling to support the hand and arm (see below), you should first make a triangular bandage. Such bandages can be bought or improvised. If you choose to make one yourself, all you need is a large square piece of linen.

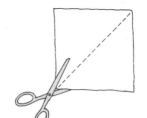
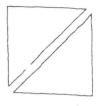

Fold a piece of linen or calico 1 m sq. diagonally in half. Cut along the fold. This makes two bandages.

Applying a Sling

Slings are used when it is necessary to afford support and protection to the upper limb. They are effective when the patient is standing or sitting. Sit the patient down comfortably and support the injured arm with the wrist and hand slightly higher than the elbow. Stand in front of the patient with a prepared triangular bandage.

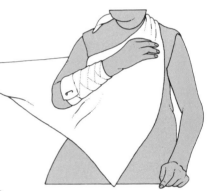

1 Place the open triangular bandage between the chest and the forearm, its point stretching well beyond the elbow.

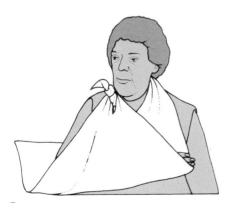

2 Carry the lower end of the bandage up and over the arm and tie off with a reef knot in front of the hollow above the collarbone on the injured side.

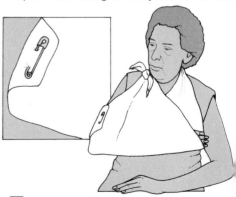

3 Bring the point forward and secure it in front of the bandage. If a safety pin is used, it should be secured vertically rather than horizontally.

BREATHING DIFFICULTIES:
Helping the patient to breathe more easily

BREATHING DIFFICULTIES

The beginning of a new life is measured from the moment when a baby takes its first breath. Breathing is vital to life. Because of this, breathing difficulties are always serious or, at the very least, disturbing for the patient. Nursing care in a large number of unrelated conditions may involve anticipating possible difficulties in breathing or relieving existing ones.

It is important to understand what happens when we breathe. Adults breathe sixteen to eighteen times a minute, and the rate increases with exercise. With each breath, air is drawn in (ideally through the nose) where it is warmed and filtered by small hairs before it passes through the pharynx and larynx, down the trachea to the lungs. The trachea is stiffened with C-shaped rings of cartilage which prevent it from collapsing. It divides and sends a branch to each lung, where it divides further into smaller and smaller air tubes (bronchioles), terminating in air sacs (alveoli). The air sacs are the spongy substance of the lungs, and it is here that oxygen passes into the blood and carbon dioxide is removed from it.

If anything interferes with the normal breathing process, breathing becomes difficult. Your task is to help the patient breathe more easily and you should therefore have some idea of what is causing the obstruction. All sorts of conditions may cause a patient to have breathing problems: a cold may block up his nose, causing him to breathe through his mouth until his throat is sore; he may inhale a crumb or a drop of liquid, making him cough until it has been expelled; he may suffer from

asthma, finding it very difficult to breathe out during an attack; or his lungs may be full of fluid, making breathing difficult, as is the case with certain categories of patients who have been confined to bed for some time.

The respiratory system

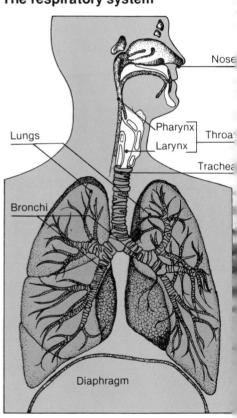

Nose

Lungs

Pharynx

Throat

Larynx

Trachea

Bronchi

Diaphragm

Helping the Patient to Breathe

For the patient to breathe easily, his air passages must be kept clear. This may be a straightforward matter of making sure he changes position frequently, or it may require some active care. The patient may have a cough that needs to be controlled,

or the asthmatic may need his spasm relieving. You may also have to help the patient to clear a blocked nose. In every case, you should assess his general condition and decide on the amount of help he needs to breathe normally.

Clearing a Blocked Nose

If the patient's upper respiratory passages are blocked or need soothing, they may be soothed and moistened with the help of steam inhalations. These are made by mixing a drug with almost boiling water and allowing the patient to inhale the vapour. (The water must be almost boiling water, not boiling, because boiling water may vapourize irritant substances as well as the soothing ones.)

Several different drugs may be mixed with the water depending on the patient's needs: friars' balsam is soothing and reduces inflammation in the trachea (tracheitis) and in the bronchi (bronchitis).

Menthol, eucalyptus and pine help to clear the air passages by shrinking the mucus membrane lining the nose and sinuses. Which drug you use, and in what quantity, will depend on the instructions given to you by the doctor or district nursing sister. In the absence of instructions, however, the normal dose is 5ml of friars' balsam to 600ml of water, or 1-2 crystals of menthol to 600ml of water.

Other methods of clearing the nose can be used: sprays can be squirted into the nose or nasal drops can be given (see page 74). Always follow the instructions on the label of such sprays and drops with care.

Giving a steam inhalation

You will need:
- a tray
- a large jug (holding 600ml)
- a thick cover for the jug
- a bowl in which to stand the jug
- water just off the boil
- the appropriate jug and a measure
- a large towel
- a sputum cup or plastic yoghurt pot (if required: see page 128)
- paper handkerchiefs.

With the patient sitting upright in bed, place a bed-table in front of him or pull a locker or table as close to the side of the bed as you can. If the patient is in a chair, place a small table in front of him. If his nose is very sore, smear the area with petroleum jelly before starting treatment.

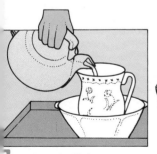 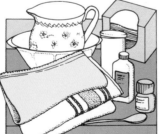 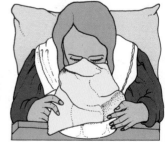

1 Pour half the water into the jug and add the drug. Add the remaining water, but **do not fill the jug more than two-thirds full.**

2 Wrap the cover around the jug and place it in the bowl on the tray, with the sputum cup and paper handkerchiefs.

3 Arrange the towel. The patient should breathe in through his mouth and out through his nose while steam rises (10-15 minutes).

Some patients prefer a bath towel over both their head and the inhaler. (Women usually prefer the method illustrated, as it is less likely to make their hair limp.)

After the treatment, clear away and leave the patient comfortable. If he is up and about, suggest that he remains in the warm for the next half hour.

Controlling the Cough

Coughing is a protective mechanism; it is the body's way of clearing the air passages. Some coughs are hard and dry while others are productive — that is to say, a great deal of mucus is coughed up (expectorated).

If the cough is hard and dry, the doctor may prescribe a linctus. This eases the pain and distress of coughing, particularly desirable at night when the patient most needs undisturbed rest. A linctus should never be diluted as the syrup-like consistency soothes the irritated passages when sipped slowly.

If there is a great deal of sputum to be coughed up, a cough mixture will be given to make the mucus thinner and easier to cough up.

All such medicines should be given according to the instructions for giving drugs on page 72.

Relieving Asthma and Hiccups

The spasm that occurs in asthma is relieved by various tablets, injections and aerosol sprays prescribed for the patient by the doctor. Make sure that they are always within the patient's reach and that he has a bell near him so that he can summon you if he has an attack. Tight clothing should be avoided, especially around the neck, as during an attack an asthmatic feels as if he is being strangled.

A child subject to regular asthmatic attacks can be taught how to use a simple inhaler or aerosol spray.

When the large muscle dividing the abdominal and chest cavities (known as the diaphragm) goes into spasm, hiccups occur. Hiccups can be extremely distressing, especially if prolonged. Sit the patient upright and try the everyday remedies: get him to hold his breath, to drink from the opposite side of a glass from the one normally held to the mouth or to blow up a paper bag. In the majority of cases, one of these methods will work. If, however, the attack is prolonged and distressing, notify the doctor.

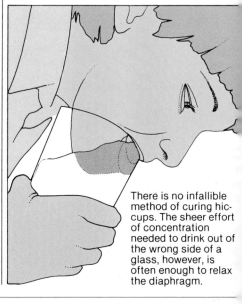

There is no infallible method of curing hiccups. The sheer effort of concentration needed to drink out of the wrong side of a glass, however, is often enough to relax the diaphragm.

Relieving Breathlessness

Various conditions cause breathlessness, which may be chronic or intermittent. The most common are severe chest and heart diseases. Before you can plan your nursing care, you should assess the patient's needs carefully. The help you give will depend on several factors: whether he is breathless all the time or only occasionally; whether breathlessness only occurs when he is walking or climbing stairs, or also when he is at rest; whether he is blue (cyanosed) or breathing more rapidly than usual. Any sudden breathlessness or change should be reported to the doctor, who will recommend treatment. What follows is general nursing care only.

Helping the Breathless Patient

Most patients with breathing difficulties find it easier to breathe when sitting upright (see page 30). A backrest and pillows will help while a board or pillow to support the feet will stop the patient slipping down the bed. This is important: if a patient with severe heart disease slips down the bed, he may, as a result, especially at night, have an attack which so closely resembles an asthmatic attack that it is known as cardiac asthma. Sometimes these patients are given a special suppository before being settled down to sleep (see page 83 for giving suppositories). The drug is absorbed from the rectum and reduces the spasm in the bronchioles.

Occasionally at home the breathless patient is nursed sitting up in an armchair. In these circumstances you must see that he changes his position regularly, and that his feet and legs are kept warm. Keep the room well ventilated at all times. Avoid giving dry foods, which will cause coughing; instead give frequent small, light meals that will tempt the appetite and reduce pressure on the diaphragm. If his air pas-

sages are dry and inflamed, a steam inhalation (see page 125) may bring relief. If he is cyanosed, oxygen may be prescribed (see page 128).

The doctor will probably ask you to observe several specific things about the breathless patient: his colour, respiratory rate and sputum.

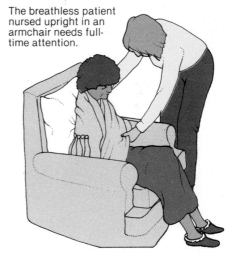

The breathless patient nursed upright in an armchair needs full-time attention.

Colour

If the patient has an infection he may be flushed. If there is insufficient oxygen in his blood he is cyanosed: his skin will have a bluish tinge, especially around the nose, mouth and the lobes of the ears. Note if the blueness is improving or not as a result of treatment, or if it is worse at any particular time of the day.

Respiratory rate

Difficulty in breathing will alter the patient's respiration and it may be necessary to count the respiratory rate (see page 105) so that the doctor can assess the effect of his treatment. This may have to be done regularly over a period of time.

Sputum

Sputum is fluid coughed up from the lungs. It varies in quantity, colour and type. Patients who produce small quantities of sputum may spit into paper handkerchiefs. Any patient with a productive cough should have a waxed carton in which to spit. At least once a day the paper handkerchiefs or carton should be placed in a plastic or paper bag and burned, or wrapped carefully in newspaper and put in the dustbin. If a carton is unobtainable, a plastic cream or yoghurt pot with a lid is an acceptable substitute.

Remember that sputum may contain bacteria and could be a source of infection. Sputum containers should, therefore, always be kept covered and should be handled carefully, especially at the time of disposal.

The doctor may ask for a specimen of sputum to be saved. If it is for laboratory examination he will supply the appropriate carton. Your duty is to make sure that the carton is clearly labelled with the patient's name, address, the date, and the nature of the contents.

Giving Oxygen

Frequently in hospital and sometimes at home a patient may be given oxygen to assist his breathing. Oxygen is supplied in a black and white cylinder. In the home a small size is used, but in hospital cylinders either stand beside the patient's bed or are stored outside the ward, the gas being conveyed to the patient along pipes set into the wall.

The oxygen is under considerable pressure inside the cylinder. Because of this, a special valve is fitted, called a reducing

valve, which prevents the gas from coming out too quickly. The amount of oxygen the patient is receiving is measured in litres per minute by a flow meter. The amount of oxygen in the cylinder is measured by a pressure gauge, indicating full, half full or quarter full.

In hospital oxygen may be given through nasal catheters, by face mask, or by placing the patient in an oxygen tent.

At home oxygen is most usually given by face mask.

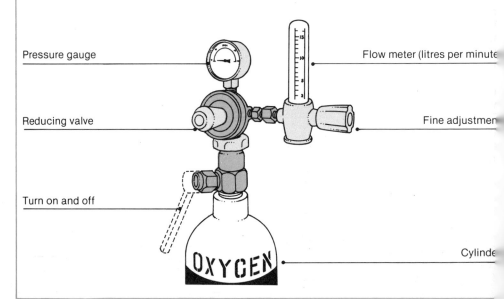

Pressure gauge

Flow meter (litres per minute

Reducing valve

Fine adjustment

Turn on and off

Cylinde

Turning on the Oxygen

Check that the cylinder is an oxygen cylinder. Read the pressure gauge to make sure the cylinder contains oxygen. Connect the apparatus to the supply, but do not yet attach it to the patient. Open the cylinder with the key and adjust the rate of flow according to your instructions (the rate is measured in litres per minute). Check that the oxygen is flowing by holding the mask near your cheek, before arranging the mask comfortably for the patient. Record the amount given in litres per minute.

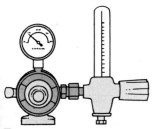

1 Check that the cylinder contains oxygen. Connect the apparatus to the supply.

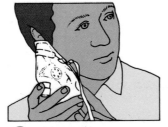

2 Open the cylinder and adjust the rate of flow. Hold the mask to your cheek to check that oxygen is flowing.

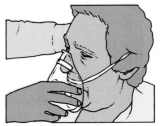

3 Place the mask over the patient's face so that it fits snugly over his nose and mouth.

Oxygen for Use in the Home

Many patients with chronic chest or heart complaints are helped by being able to breathe oxygen when climbing stairs or moving about. In these cases, the family doctor will refer the patient to a consultant, who can prescribe the most suitable apparatus, which the hospital will then lend to the patient and maintain.

There are several makes of portable oxygen cylinder available, each supplied with a shoulder strap and carrying bag. They weigh between 2.5 and 5kg each and hold from 100 to 500 litres of oxygen. The patient is also supplied with a gauge and a face mask.

Portable cylinders can be filled from an ordinary oxygen cylinder, with the help of a special recharging adaptor. No special skill is needed and the procedure takes about twelve minutes. Many chemists now operate a while-you-wait refill service, in which case the family doctor may prescribe the refill cylinder.

Other more sophisticated or elegant pieces of equipment, apart from the ones that are available through the National Health Service, may be bought, but these are all very expensive.

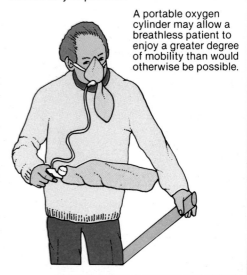

A portable oxygen cylinder may allow a breathless patient to enjoy a greater degree of mobility than would otherwise be possible.

Dangers of Oxygen

Whether oxygen is used at home or in an institution, the dangers are the same. No naked light or spark (such as from a mechanical toy) must be allowed to come anywhere near oxygen: fire spreads with frightening rapidity in the presence of this gas. Smoking is strictly forbidden: a glowing cigarette will burst into flames.

Grease or oil should not be used on the valve or flow meter, nor should these be touched with greasy hands. Grease and oil may ignite spontaneously in the presence of oxygen, causing an explosion.

If you remember these three things when dealing with oxygen, you should be safe:
- no sparks
- no smoking
- no grease

Caring for a Tracheostomy

An increasing number of patients breathe through an artificial opening in the neck called a tracheostomy. You should be aware of the reasons for this if you are to care for the patient adequately.

The operation is carried out when there is an obstruction to breathing like a growth in the voice box (larynx) or, more rarely, because of severe flame or caustic burns. As a temporary measure, unconscious patients being nursed in an intensive care unit or patients with severe respiratory problems may be artificially ventilated through a tracheostomy. In these cases, however, when the patient is better the tube is removed and the opening heals.

In the early stages of all types of tracheostomy a tube is inserted through the hole into the trachea, but this is sometimes discarded later. Should you be helping to care for a patient who has had a tracheostomy, as part of your daily care you will have to look after his tube. This is particularly important if he has a chest infection, as mucus can clog up the tube and obstruct his breathing. Ask the patient or a relative how the tube is normally cleaned and follow their instructions. In the absence of any instructions, rinse the tube either under running water or in bicarbonate of soda solution (one 5ml spoonful of bicarbonate of soda to 600ml of water). Rinse it well before returning it to the patient for use.

If the patient's voice box has been removed he will be unable to talk. Some people are taught by a speech therapist to belch air from the stomach and make sounds, others never achieve this skill. If the voice box is still there, a little valve in the tracheostomy tube closes when the patient wishes to speak. Anticipate his problem by making sure that you have pencil and paper to hand.

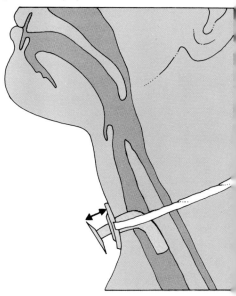

A tracheostomy is an easy operation, which may be performed under either a general or a local anaesthetic. A tube is inserted to open an air passage between the trachea and the front of the neck when the throat or larynx is blocked. The tracheostomy may be temporary or permanent.

COMMUNICATION:
Helping the patient to communicate his needs effectively

COMMUNICATION

Communication is an essential social process. People need to communicate: to express their anxieties and their emotions, to make known their wants, and to go about their daily lives. As a volunteer you should be sensitive to all the ways in which a patient may try and communicate, whether these are verbal or non-verbal. In certain illnesses where the patient has difficulties in making his needs known, what little verbal communication there is may be especially important, while non-verbal communication forms the basis for many observations.

Non-Verbal Communication

Animals exist entirely without the spoken word. They make friends, find mates, rear young, establish their territories and co-operate in groups using only expressions, posture, gesture, smell, and noises. Much human communication is also non-verbal. A person's facial expression reveals if he is happy or angry. A sagging posture suggests weariness, dejection or unhappiness. The outstretched arms of the mother promise love and security. A handshake is a mark of introduction and acceptance; in some business circles it acts as a bond. Movements of the head may denote agreement or disapproval. From earliest childhood we are taught to recognize these signs and many others. Learning to be sensitive to them is part of learning to live in society.

It is not difficult to apply your knowledge of people in general to the patient. When entering a patient's room you observe his face: he may look tense, totally blank, or have a face screwed up with pain. Caught unobserved, the weary or dejected person slumps in the bed or chair, the depressed person tends to huddle in a corner, and the person with a headache lies with his face turned away from the light or with his hands covering his eyes. The person with abdominal pain tends to lie on his side and draw up his legs. The frightened person grips your hand or arm, the frustrated child bangs his head against the side of his cot and the agitated elderly person mutters to himself. These signs of the patient's feelings are all relatively obvious; the better you know an individual patient, the more easily you will come to recognize non-verbal signals far more subtle than these.

The three patients here are all communicating
— either boredom, apathy, or total dejection.

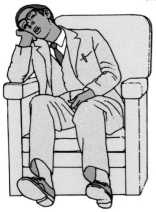 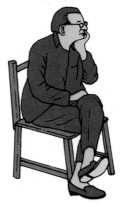 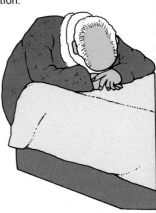

Verbal Communication

Verbal communication is fully as important as non-verbal. If you cannot understand another person because of a speech impediment or the inability to speak his language, you cannot exchange ideas or share experiences. Communication is reduced to exaggerated gestures and mime. It is like shopping abroad when you do not speak the language. Most people just point to the article they want or make gestures to explain it. On the whole this proves successful: when language fails, it is acceptable to fall back on mime.

Unless English is not the patient's mother tongue, verbal communication only presents a problem if disease or damage have interfered with the normal speech processes.

Communication Problems

One of the main difficulties experienced by voluntary workers is an uncertainty as to how to approach the patient, whether his disability is physical or emotional. This can be overcome by obtaining help and advice from the district nursing sister, health visitor or specialist social worker. Be sensitive to the needs of the patient and anticipate his wants. Try and understand how his particular condition is affecting his ability to communicate. Be patient and give him the time and opportunity to express his wants and feelings. If you have no other time to set aside, often during a blanket bath or other similar procedure there is the opportunity and the time to encourage the patient to talk.

Always address yourself directly to the patient, even if he cannot answer you and even if he is handicapped. Some people have the habit of talking as if the patient were not present. They address his companion to say "Well, how is he today?" Imagine how frustrated you would be if you were the patient. Even if he cannot respond, include him in the conversation. Talk about your leisure activities, or any subject that will give him interest and pleasure. This is especially important if the patient is confined to one room.

The Patient Who Cannot Talk

The patient may be unable to talk (aphasic) as the result of a stroke. His hearing is not affected and he knows what he wants, but he cannot tell you. Some patients can speak, but are incapable of saying the right word; after much effort they come out with a word that is quite inappropriate. This causes further distress.

Quite literally these patients have to be taught to speak again. This requires patience on your part, and perseverance on the part of the patient. A speech therapist will assess the patient and commence treatment, but she cannot be with him all the time, so there is a lot of scope for relatives, friends and volunteers to help. In the early stages picture cards can be useful: when the patient has an obvious need that he cannot express you show him a selection of picture cards. These may be made with pictures from magazines. He can then point to the bedpan or glass of water that he needs.

Another group of patients deprived of speech are those who have had their voice box (larynx) removed. Some of these patients are eventually taught to speak again, but it is a long and difficult process. However successful the result, the patient's speech can never sound like a normal voice. All you can do for these patients is to offer constant encouragement and support, so that they are motivated towards speech.

The Deaf Patient

The deaf patient's inability to hear makes it hard for him to communicate. If, as is common among the elderly, hearing fails gradually, the patient often accuses other people of mumbling: he begins to feel isolated and rejected. He may even become suspicious and feel that people are talking about him and laughing at him when in fact they are just taking part in an ordinary conversation. A hearing aid may help: remember, however, that a hearing aid magnifies *all* sounds, including background noise, and so it is not always as useful as it might seem. Plenty of non-verbal signs and a specialist to teach lip-reading may be more helpful.

A little thought in the early stages of deafness can serve to minimize the sense of isolation. Never turn your back on a deaf person while talking to him. Try and use the lower tones of your voice range as these are more readily heard. Include the person in your smiles and gestures when possible.

Because deafness often leads to a very restricted social life there is scope for much welfare work among the deaf. It is a field in which the voluntary organizations offer a great deal of help.

The Blind Patient

The blind patient can talk and can hear, but non-verbal communication is largely inaccessible to him. You cannot hear a smile or an outstretched hand. Blindness may result from injury, it may accompany another disease or it may come as part of the ageing process. Once the initial shock wears off the patient has to adapt to a new way of life. His hearing and sense of touch must develop, he may learn braille and other new skills. Some patients adapt readily and others do not. Ageing often brings a gradual loss of sight, allowing time for some adaptation to occur during the partially sighted period. This group of patients often need special understanding and support: hearing may be failing at the same time as sight, while simultaneously patients are often becoming less active and mobile.

Deafness and blindness in childhood

The deaf child Deafness is virtually impossible to diagnose in the newborn baby, who does not react to sounds in a predictable way. A deaf baby under six months old will make babbling noises just like a normal baby. But it is essential to diagnose deafness early in order to make use of every scrap of hearing the child may have: it is by imitation of sounds heard that the child learns to talk and so communicate with others. Doctors and health visitors working in child health clinics therefore pay special attention to hearing tests. Even a six-month-old baby can be fitted with a hearing aid and so learn to interpret sounds.

Deaf children attend special schools where no effort is spared to teach them the art of communication. Hearing aids, microphones, lip reading, mime, sign language and machines which reproduce sound as patterns of light are all used to this end.

The blind child Total blindness at birth is not common, but a number of children have sight defects serious enough to necessitate special attention at school. The totally blind infant usually goes to a residential nursery school, where he is trained to move about in an independent way. His education continues at a special school, with emphasis on teaching by sound and the use of braille for reading.

The Non-English Speaking Patient

Patients whose first language is not English may have difficulty in communicating unrelated to any physical impairment. Often they have the additional disadvantage of being unfamiliar with English culture and the English way of life. Women in particular often become severely depressed with no contact outside their own family; relatives may need to be persuaded to allow them to visit a doctor. Cultural influence must be respected: for instance, some Moslem women are reluctant to undress, particularly if they are to be examined by a male doctor.

Try and communicate with these patients somehow, whether it be through another member of the family or an interpreter. Try also to arrange for these patients to meet and talk with other people who speak their language, and to join in social activities with them. The more frequently you attend to someone in this position, the more easily you will understand the patient's needs, and the easier the patient will find it to transmit emotions and fears. As a practical measure, language cards (available from the Red Cross) may help you get the answer to questions.

The Confused Patient

Temporary confusion may occur if a patient has a high temperature or is suffering from mental illness. Most confused patients, however, belong to the older age groups. A confused patient may not know where he is, what day of the week it is or what he wants. He may wander about in a dazed way and do potentially dangerous things. Always make sure the doctor knows if a patient is confused as all types of patient may benefit from some medical treatment.

Confusion associated with infection

When the patient has an infection, confusion may arise from the toxic state and from the dehydration caused by the raised temperature. Replacement of the fluid and reduction of the temperature bring a speedy improvement.

Confusion in the elderly

The elderly often become confused when they are moved to different surroundings, to hospital, for instance. Not uncommonly in these circumstances they cling to a particular nurse or volunteer, insisting that she is their daughter, niece or long-lost friend. Something in the appearance or

manner of the individual probably triggers off a memory and the association is made. The confusion is often lessened if the number of people involved in the patient's general care is reduced; adding vitamin B to the diet and improving the patient's general health are also beneficial.

If the patient's sight or hearing are impaired the problem is increased. Much patience is needed among those caring for this group and repeated explanations of the simplest things may be needed.

Confusion in the mentally ill

Confusion from mental illness may arise as a result of the illness itself or of the treatment given. If you want to communicate with the mentally ill, it is not just a matter of establishing contact with the patient, but also the difficulty of overcoming barriers within yourself. People are often over-anxious and even frightened of mental illness, and do not know how or where to begin to help the patient with his difficulties.

Volunteers who are caring for the mentally ill often ask: "What should I say?" There is no magic formula, no easy answer, but with care and thought it is unlikely that anything you do or say will be harmful to the patient. If in doubt, try listening rather than talking.

Helping the Mentally Ill

Listening is often of great value. Many patients are able to unburden themselves of great misery simply by talking to a sympathetic listener who is not too busy to listen. Sit quietly, give the patient your undivided attention and you may find that you only need to smile or nod and he will be encouraged to continue. If he does not talk, just sit with him in a companionable silence. This is very comforting and is often appreciated, as the patient feels he matters to someone.

Just as the patient's spiritual adviser brings help and comfort in physical illness, he may also be of help in a mental illness. If the patient wishes it, inform the relevant person and give him the opportunity to visit. Both the patient and his family may benefit. You may also benefit: his knowledge of the patient, his family, their cultural and spiritual background and religious or national customs may prove very useful.

The patient in the community

The patient being cared for in the community needs the support of his family, his employer and all those around him. They must accept him as he is, realizing that the behaviour which seems odd or irrational to them is quite rational to him. All he says and does is affected by his illness.

The patient who has been in hospital

If the patient's condition required his admission to hospital his subsequent return home is often effected gradually. First he goes home for weekends and then, as he improves, for longer periods, until his final discharge. Once home he may still require help and support, so he and his family will be visited regularly either by some of the team who cared for him in hospital or their community counterpart.

Sometimes the transition from hospital to home is too difficult and the patient may go first into a special hostel. This is a half-way house. From the hostel he goes to work, visits his family and friends, but has expert support when he needs it. When his self-confidence has returned he can finally resume life at home.

The majority of patients spend less than six weeks in hospital, but a return to full health takes longer than this. The majority are cured quite quickly. Some take longer, but only a few are incurable.

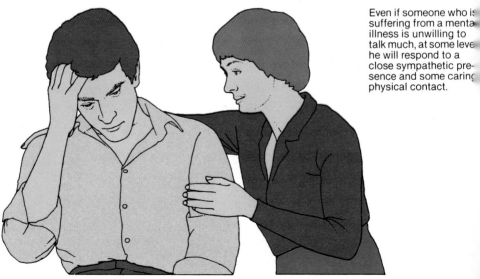

Even if someone who is suffering from a mental illness is unwilling to talk much, at some level he will respond to a close sympathetic presence and some caring physical contact.

RECOVERY AND REHABILITATION:
Helping the patient towards complete recovery

RECOVERY AND REHABILITATION

Pressure on National Health Service beds means that patients are now being discharged from hospital as early as possible into the care of the family practitioner and the district nursing sister. As a volunteer you may well be asked to help care for such patients.

You may also be caring for day patients in the home: these include patients who regularly attend hospital for treatment, daily or less often for short periods; and patients who attend a centre for the whole day from Monday to Friday. It will help you to know what is happening to them during this time.

Patients Newly Discharged from Hospital

When a patient is discharged from hospital into the home, you will need information on a number of points in order to assess his condition and estimate how much and what sort of care he needs.
- How much activity may he undertake?
- How much rest should he have?
- Are there medicines to be given?
- Are there arrangements for dressings to be changed or stitches removed?
- Has he an outpatient appointment?
- When may he return to work?

It is a great temptation for a patient to think that, once he is home, he is absolutely fit and can do anything. The housewife particularly tends to come home and take over the household duties at once. In fact, the newly discharged patient tires easily, as he is always much weaker than he suspected when pottering round the ward. In spite of his eagerness to get home, he is often restless and depressed, finding it hard to settle down. He is missing the security of the hospital ward. Tolerance and understanding help the patient through this phase of recovery.

All convalescent patients, irrespective of age, should be encouraged to rest for at least an hour every afternoon, preferably on the bed where they can really relax. To allow for enough rest, domestic help may be needed. If the members of the family cannot provide this, private help or a home help should be suggested. The Social Services department provide a home help

service where it is needed, with the patient paying according to his income.

All patients need to take exercise, and the doctor will guide you about the amount. Plenty of fluids and an interesting diet appetizingly served will also promote recovery. The patient may need help with shopping and the provision of meals. Neighbours, the home help and young people in voluntary organizations are often willing to help with the shopping, while the Meals on Wheels service may be able to provide a midday meal (see p. 64).

Your nursing care and the advice you give will obviously depend on the patient's condition. The patient recovering from an abdominal operation, for instance, should avoid lifting and carrying. Certain patients have special needs. These may be practical, psychological or both. If the patient has had an operation such as a mastectomy, for instance, she will need practical help in choosing a suitable prosthesis but above all she will be in need of psychological support. If a treatment such as a dressing or injection is required, the district nursing sister will visit. She will tell the family if there is any equipment she would like provided for her use. If a patient is being discharged from hospital at a weekend or Bank holiday, it is essential to make sure that the hospital provides an adequate number of dressings for use until a prescription can be obtained from the doctor and dispensed by the chemist.

The Convalescent Child

A child needs special understanding after a stay in hospital, even if one or both parents have been able to stay with him for most of the time. The unfamiliarity of hospital surroundings combine with any pain or uncomfortable procedures to disturb the child and make him feel insecure. For a while after his return home, especially if the stay has been a long one, the child may behave as if he were younger than his years. This is known as regressive behaviour and it may take many different forms: the exploring toddler may become clinging and shy, the child competent at feeding herself may revert to bottles, and the child dry for over a year may start wetting his pants. If the family and all those caring for the child offer love, security and understanding, the child will gradually regain his normal level of development.

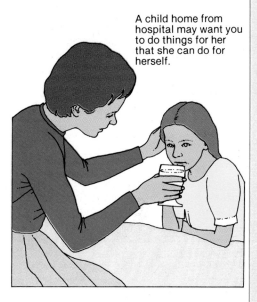

A child home from hospital may want you to do things for her that she can do for herself.

The New Mother

The mother with a new baby is tired and anxious. A demanding baby is causing broken nights and generally disturbing the household. Often the most tiring aspect of the newborn baby's behaviour is its unpredictability. Until a few weeks have passed and the baby has settled into a pattern, the mother can never be sure what the baby is going to do next. She cannot be immediately sure why he is crying, whether he is still hungry or if he is sleeping enough.

In these circumstances the new mother should be offered as much help and support as possible. If she can be encouraged to remain calm, she will communicate a relaxed feeling to her baby, who will respond by settling more quickly. The domiciliary or home midwife usually visits the mother and baby at home for ten days after the birth, with the health visitor taking over on the eleventh day. If there is any anxiety about the mother — particularly if she seems depressed or the baby is not well — contact the midwife, health visitor or family doctor as soon as possible.

A mother getting to know her new baby needs to be given plenty of time to relax and adjust to the change in her way of life.

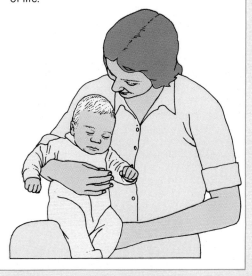

Day Patients

People who attend hospitals or centres as day patients may do so for a variety of different reasons. Patients attending hospital may be receiving continuous daily treatment or they may be attending regularly, but intermittently, for a specific course of therapy. Patients attending a centre may also receive treatment, but this is likely to be combined with social activities. Some centres provide only a social service.

Treatments at Day Hospitals

Radiotherapy

This consists of special X-rays, which destroy unwanted tissue while leaving the surrounding tissue undamaged. A course of treatment may last from four to six weeks and leave the patient very weak. Nausea is not uncommon and the patient is often reluctant to eat.

The skin over the treatment area may become red and sore, particularly if it is an area where sweating and friction occur, such as the armpit or the skin under the breast. The patient will be given very detailed instructions on how to care for the area and these must be followed exactly, as many soaps, powders and creams only aggravate the condition.

As treatment continues, weakness and tiredness increase and vomiting and diarrhoea may occur. Morale is low. The patient — already apprehensive because of his disease — feels the treatment is having no effect. Encouragement and support are vital at this stage. As a volunteer, you may well be familiar with the patient's symptoms: they are the result of radiation and are a less severe manifestation of those seen in radiation sickness caused by nuclear activity. The difference is that the patient is receiving *controlled* doses of radiation: when the treatment stops the symptoms will disappear. Offer reassurance along these lines.

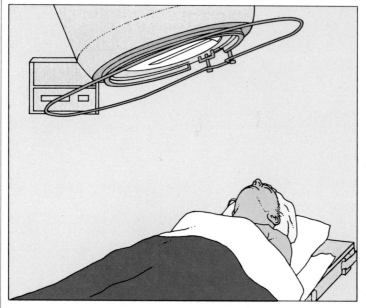

Radiotherapy consists of controlled doses of radiation aimed at a precisely defined part of the body. The treatment does not hurt at all, but precautions are taken so that radiation cannot penetrate areas other than the one needing treatment. Cancer is not the only condition for which radiotherapy is used; some patients may derive great reassurance from this.

Physiotherapy

This is given for many muscular and joint conditions. It is also used to re-educate limbs that have been immobilized after surgery or fracture, and limbs weakened after a stroke. Exercises are often taught as part of the treatment and the patient may need encouragement and assistance to persevere.

Patients having regular physiotherapy or radiotherapy often need transport; they may be able to use the hospital car service.

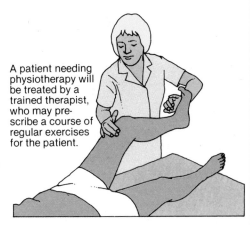

A patient needing physiotherapy will be treated by a trained therapist, who may prescribe a course of regular exercises for the patient.

Attendance at Day Centres

Day centres have been established in many areas. Handicapped and elderly patients are collected by ambulance or voluntary transport in the morning and taken to a centre (which may or may not be in a hospital) where they spend the day. Here there may be facilities for physiotherapy, hydrotherapy and occupational therapy. The patients are also given a well-balanced midday meal. Social activities are often included, so the patients are kept occupied all day; they return home in the evening.

The voluntary organizations are actively concerned in the work of many of the day centres. They may fetch patients and take them home, organize social activities, and offer nursing care if necessary, such as bathing or feeding patients. In many cases, without the help of volunteers it would be impossible to staff day centres adequately.

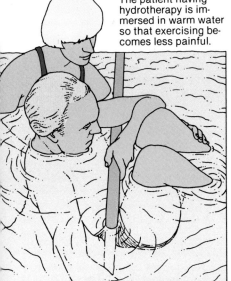

The patient having hydrotherapy is immersed in warm water so that exercising becomes less painful.

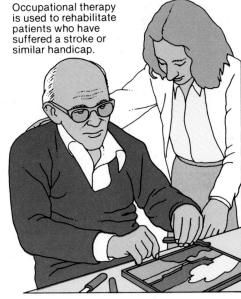

Occupational therapy is used to rehabilitate patients who have suffered a stroke or similar handicap.

Outpatients

Whereas day patients usually attend hospital for post-operative treatment, outpatients most commonly attend for pre-operative investigations.

It is impossible to mention all the reasons why someone may have to attend the outpatient department, but a little knowledge about some of the more common ones may prove useful.

Plaster of paris

Patients with a fractured limb, particularly an upper limb, have plaster of paris applied and are then sent home. While the plaster is drying, avoid direct heat and support the part comfortably on a pillow. There is a danger that the injured limb may swell inside the plaster and cause constriction, so if the patient feels increasing pain in the limbs, if the fingers or toes look blue, swollen or feel cold, it is advisable to take him back to the hospital.

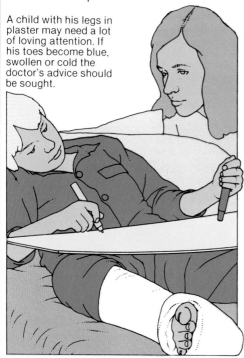

A child with his legs in plaster may need a lot of loving attention. If his toes become blue, swollen or cold the doctor's advice should be sought.

Dilatation and curettage (D & C)

A dilatation and curettage is a scraping of the womb (uterus), done to examine the womb lining when the patient has suffered excessive or irregular bleeding. Afterwards there is likely to be a heavier blood loss than during a menstrual period, but after 24 hours this should begin to decrease. Encourage the patient to take it easy until the bleeding has stopped.

Barium X-ray

Barium is a substance which shows up on an X-ray film. It is given by mouth to line the stomach when there is a gastric complaint, and X-rays may be taken at specified intervals to follow the progress of the barium through the small and large intestine and discover any abnormality. Barium may also be given as an enema.

A day or two before the investigation, the patient may be given tablets to take. These are usually to empty the rectum and reduce the gas in the intestine. Because barium is white, following the investigation the patient will pass white stools. He may also be constipated for a day or two.

Gastroscopy

Gastroscopy also investigates stomach conditions. A flexible tube is passed through the mouth into the stomach. With the help of a light and a series of mirrors, the doctor is able to look at the stomach lining. Patients often complain of a sore throat and have difficulty in swallowing for a day or two after gastroscopy.

Cystoscopy

Cystoscopy is a similar investigation: the tube is passed into the bladder. It is common for the patient to experience discomfort when passing urine for 24 hours after the investigation. Blood may also be passed with the urine. Encourage the patient to drink plenty of fluids as this helps to prevent infection and makes it easier to pass urine.

RECREATIONAL ACTIVITIES:
Helping the patient to make good use of his time

RECREATIONAL ACTIVITIES

Recreation means exactly what it says: re-creation. It covers any activity that is found to be refreshing and renewing. Patients need it as much as anybody else, but many find it almost impossible to think up or to arrange for themselves.

As a volunteer you have a very special part to play in helping with recreational activities. You may just be concerned with the needs of one patient in the home; on the other hand, many volunteers visit hospitals and homes for the elderly or disabled to talk with patients, write their letters and play games with them. Others are asked to help with group activities such as sing-songs and outings. Their involvement is invaluable not only for the patients but for those who staff the homes and hospitals.

Planning Recreation

Recreation must be carefully planned and designed to suit the patient's particular need. The better you know an individual, the more accurately you will be able to tailor your suggestions to his need, but there are several general points to consider.

Much will depend on the patient's age and sex as well as his health. Most impor-tant, what are his interests and what facilities are available for him to pursue them? If his illness has imposed any limitations — mental or physical — on his ability to pursue his interest, these should be considered. In certain cases it may be possible to combine recreation with the patient's rehabilitation.

Stages of Illness

The amount of time during the day that the patient has to spend on recreation and the enthusiasm he displays will partly depend on the stage of his illness.

At the height of his illness the patient will tire easily and his powers of concentration may be reduced. Even at this stage planning some recreation into his day will help to counteract the debility and depression felt during and after an illness.

Radio and television demand no physical activity and every effort should be made to avoid meals or nursing care during the patient's favourite programmes. Many housebound people find comfort in participating in broadcast religious services. Many men are football or cricket fanatics, while others enjoy boxing or racing. If the patient loves music, and a record-player is available, put on his favourite records; if he is in hospital enquire if the hospital broadcasts a request programme on its own wavelength. Make sure that the television is properly adjusted and the radio or record-player are not too loud. If the patient cannot reach the controls, be available to switch off when he tires.

Even patients who can hardly move because of weakness or paralysis can derive a great deal of pleasure from bird life. Hang a nut basket or piece of fat near the patient's window and keep the bird table stocked with bread and seeds. An extra-ordinary number and variety of birds will be attracted to it. These patients may also take pleasure in watching a few fish in a bowl. They may appreciate a change of picture on the walls; these can often be borrowed from a local picture library.

To enjoy reading, the patient must be capable of more concentration. The short articles of a magazine or newspaper may be easier for him to absorb than the more demanding length of a book. If the patient has no specific preferences, consult the local librarian and try and get hold of some art books or travel books with more pictures than text. These are often of interest to the patient, especially if you can chat together about places you have visited. If his sight is poor, try and borrow the special large print books from the library.

Remember that all large books are heavy and the patient may need to prop them up against a bed table or a pillow.

For the totally blind there are talking books: these are specially recorded readings supplied with a machine to play them. A wide range of fiction and non-fiction is available. Some areas even have a local talking newspaper available weekly or monthly with all the local news.

Many women, and some men, may be interested in knitting, crochet or needlework. If they want something new, you might suggest they try macrame work. A walk round a good handicraft shop will keep you up to date with new ideas.

Some patients may be attracted by jigsaw or crossword puzzles; others may be stimulated to draw or paint. The patient will probably enjoy a game of cards, chess or scrabble if a friend can be persuaded to drop in for an hour or so.

People in hospital eagerly await the trolley shop to buy writing paper, soap and other small necessities. The house-bound can derive the same pleasure from shopping by post. This allows them to choose things for themselves and to plan small surprises for other members of the family at birthdays and Christmas.

Activities for the Convalescent

As convalescence progresses and the patient begins to be up and about, a walk in the garden to see the flowers and the vegetables creates an interest and a sense of achievement. The keen gardener will enjoy gardening programmes on radio and television and will gladly read gardening books, but even more, he will appreciate a vase of flowers from his own garden or an indoor plant to tend. The elderly or handicapped may be able to continue gardening if a flower-bed is raised or they are supplied with a suitable kneeler and light tools.

After a long illness a walk as far as the pillar-box or round the block is a tremendous boost to the patient's morale. A short car ride can also be very pleasant, especially if the driver uses a little imagination.

If patients are severely handicapped or need activities to get stiff limbs moving again, the occupational therapist will give help and advice. You only have to think of the Olympic Games for the disabled to see what can be achieved in spite of difficulties. At the same time you should be realistic: just as most ordinary people are unlikely to compete in the Olympics, most of your patients will not reach Olympic

standard either. The important thing, in this as in all recreational activities, is to capture their interest and relieve the tedium of illness for a short period. If you are successful in this aim, all the energy you put into planning activities will be well worthwhile.

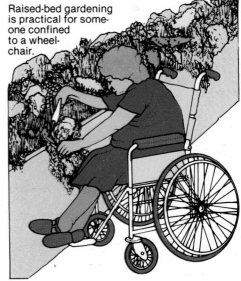

Raised-bed gardening is practical for someone confined to a wheelchair.

Planning Activities for Children

Children pose a special problem. When they are very ill they are not interested in much except perhaps a favourite toy to cuddle or a story. But as soon as a child begins to feel better he is easily bored and needs constant attention. Keeping him occupied becomes difficult, particularly if he has an infectious disease and cannot play with friends or brothers and sisters.

A convalescent child confined to bed will not stay quiet beneath the bedclothes. Because his movements in and on the bed will disturb the bedclothes, he will stay much warmer if he is dressed.

If you are buying toys, give the child one or two small ones every day rather than a big toy expected to engross him for the length of his illness. This way every day will bring him something new and relieve the monotony — especially important in sickness when you cannot expect the child to concentrate for long.

Lego and jigsaw puzzles are very popular. But if you are giving the child puzzles or games, start with an easy one and progress to something more suited to his age as he gets better: a sick child is likely to give up in frustration and misery if he cannot do a

puzzle, whereas the same child when well would have the determination to carry on trying until successful.

Small doses of radio and television may be relaxing for a child confined to bed. Make sure that you are at hand to turn the set on or off and to change channels if the child is not allowed out of bed.

Drawing and painting are much enjoyed by children in bed. Even quite small children can be successfully occupied for long periods in colouring picture books. If you are encouraging messy activities, do make sure that both the child and the bed are protected: an old sheet is very useful for this. If the child is painting give him a pot with very little water placed on a tray; if the water spills it will stay on the tray.

Try and make a game out of nursing care and tell stories while you are bathing the child or carrying out treatments. Above all, remember that ill children need even more love and attention than usual. Take time to give the child a special cuddle, especially at the end of the day when he may be restless, hot and tired. Sit him on your knee to read a story: this is one of the best ways to soothe a restless child to sleep.

A child whose reading ability is normally good may nevertheless prefer to leaf through a picture book with his mother when he is feeling unwell and his concentration is poor.

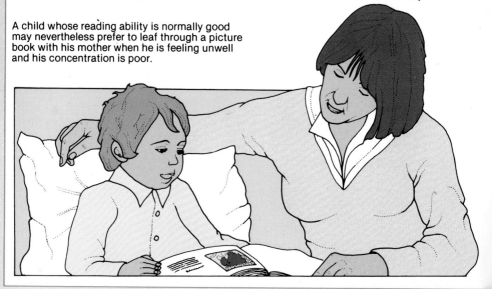

LEARNING AND RE-LEARNING:
Helping the patient to overcome disabilities and master new skills

LEARNING AND RE-LEARNING

A baby at birth knows nothing about the world. To develop normally he must learn. The only way he can learn is by taking an interest in his surroundings. For this reason every healthy baby is born curious.

Curiosity is an important factor in child development. Without it the infant would not begin to explore his world: feeling, tasting and touching the things around him, trying to find out more about them. As he grows he begins to crawl or shuffle about and eventually he walks. His new mobility enables him to make new discoveries. When he becomes able to use and understand language, he is well on the way to making sense of the world.

Every mother watches her child pass through these stages towards independence with delight and some anxiety. The young child has no sense of danger and risks injuring himself. He must be watched constantly, yet he must be allowed to be adventurous. Exploring and finding out are vital to his development.

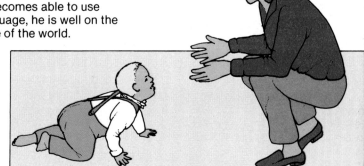

Every stage of a normal child's development is met by a loving mother with enthusiasm, encouragement — and some trepidation. Each step towards mobility brings its dangers as well as its triumphs.

Difficulties with Learning

If his basic needs for food, exercise, fresh air and shelter are met and if he is surrounded by love and affection, the healthy child develops normally. Sometimes, however, mental or physical handicap interferes with the process of development. Although handicapped children are usually still curious, because of their disability their ability to learn is impaired.

A certain number of children are born with a physical disability, while in others a handicap develops later as the result of illness or injury. The handicap itself may vary from a minor disorder of function to some major disability which can never be completely overcome. The blind or deaf child, for instance, has lost one of his vital aids to recovery. Whatever the handicap, the aim of care is the same: to allow the child to live as full and as active a life as possible, while maintaining his self-respect and encouraging his independence.

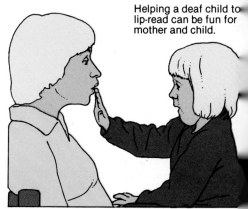

Helping a deaf child to lip-read can be fun for mother and child.

Some children fail to progress in their development because of a mental handicap. Many such children seem curious but do not seem able to learn normally. Their mental age is far below their age in years and accordingly their behaviour is that of a younger child.

Mentally handicapped children are often loving and affectionate, but their presence in a family often imposes a great emotional strain. Families in this position should call on the support and advice of professional workers, so that they can be helped to build up reserves of love and patience.

With love and patience even the severely handicapped child can usually learn simple skills. He may be able to feed and dress himself and carry out simple, repetitive tasks. However limited his potential, he must be helped to develop it to the full.

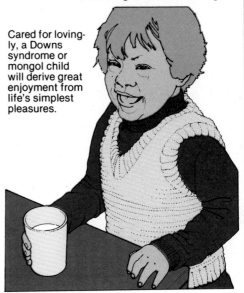

Cared for lovingly, a Downs syndrome or mongol child will derive great enjoyment from life's simplest pleasures.

The Need to Re-Learn

In certain circumstances following an illness or an accident an adult may have to re-learn many things. Just as natural curiosity in a child should be encouraged, in an adult it may have to be re-awakened, so that he may discover what he can do and gain enough confidence to extend himself further still. The patient who has had a stroke, for example, may have to learn to speak again, to feed himself with only one hand and chew his food with a part of his face which he cannot control. He may have to learn to walk with a paralysed leg and struggle to re-learn many simple skills he mastered as a young child.

The man who has lost an arm in an accident not only has to master the skills of everyday living but may have to be retrained at his old job or learn to do a new one. The patient with spinal damage must learn to propel a wheelchair, re-learn the skills of driving with hand controls and adapt his daily living to wheelchair height. These are just some examples of circumstances making re-learning necessary.

To be successful in cases of severe handicap physical re-education requires a team approach. The detailed planning is for the expert, but each professional worker and volunteer contributes his own special skills. The patient's family and his friends can all help in giving the care. In some cases progress is slow, while too much physical activity is damaging. You should be aware of this, and stay in close contact with the experts, so that you can consult with them before giving any care.

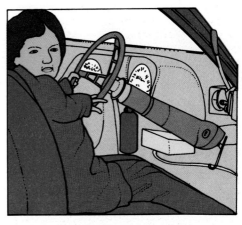

Sophisticated aids enable someone born without developed limbs to drive a car successfully.

The Need to Modify Skills

When the day of retirement comes it brings a loss of friends and a change in status. Income is often severely reduced. Unless they have a wide range of interests, retired people risk finding themselves lonely and bored. Because of this it is worthwhile planning activities for retirement in some detail beforehand. People who have devoted time to thinking about how they are going to fill their days often come to find retirement a period of great fulfilment, when at last they are able to indulge in all the pursuits they did not have time to try when they were working.

Many people turn to their garden or take up golf. Others find satisfaction in the abundance of day and evening classes run by the local education authority (where senior citizens are often entitled to pay reduced fees). Such classes provide companionship, interest and the opportunity to learn something new.

As the years pass, however, even the most contented and fulfilled people usually find that they have to modify or re-learn skills. The normal ageing process causes the eyes to dim, hearing to lose its clarity, and people to become generally slower. Bones are brittle and break more easily,

The range of sporting activities open to retired people is greater than they perhaps imagine.

while mobility may also be affected. The sense of smell is less acute, so that smoke or escaping gas, for instance, may go unnoticed. All or some of these gradually encroaching disabilities may eventually cause the patient to need nursing care and attention.

An elderly person living on her own should be visited at least daily — perhaps by a friend dropping in with some shopping for a cup of tea.

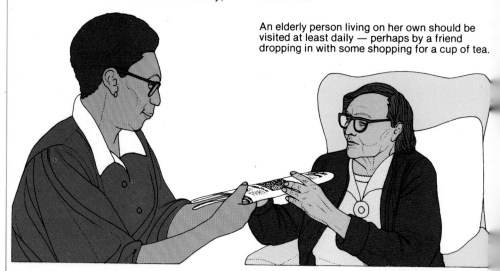

THE PATIENT WHO IS DYING:
Helping the patient to a peaceful and dignified death

THE PATIENT WHO IS DYING

Caring for the dying is no easy task. It calls for the exercise of technical skill supported by compassion and imagination. When approached for the first time, it is often very frightening. But it can also bring deep satisfaction to those providing the care, in spite of the demands made on time, physical strength and patience.

Death comes in many forms: sometimes so suddenly that no care is possible; sometimes unexpectedly during an acute illness; more often as the expected end of a long and sometimes painful illness. Many patients in the last category may come to know or suspect that they are dying and they may wish to be cared for in their own homes. While relatives feel they should agree to this, they are often anxious that they may not be able to cope and give the patient the care and support that he needs. The problems involved should therefore be listed and faced so that those providing the care can appreciate what is required.

If you are caring for someone who is dying you should be prepared to:
• cope with feelings and fears about death, both your own and the patient's
• know how to make the patient comfortable
• recognize the signs of approaching death
• know what to do when death comes.

Feelings and Fears about Death

When a patient has been ill for some weeks and it becomes apparent that his general condition is deteriorating, he tires quickly, cannot make the effort he used to and often loses weight.

At this stage the question arises as to what the patient should be told about his illness. There is no easy answer. Much depends on the patient himself. He may know that he is dying and he may not need to ask anyone for the truth. He may ask someone just to seek confirmation of what he already knows. On the other hand he may ask the newest, least experienced person involved in his care "Am I going to get better?" or "Am I dying?", knowing that because of her inexperience and lack of knowledge she cannot give him the answer he does not want to hear.

Many people hesitate to talk about death. This is, perhaps, because it is the common experience we all face and yet one of which we have a limited knowledge. But at some time in our lives we all experience grief and loss. It may be the loss of a toy, a friendship, a home or a loved one; it may be the loss of a limb. As we grow older more of our friends die and we come to realize our own mortality. Grief is the reaction to our loss and the process by which we inwardly accept the reality of an event that has already occurred. It is the process by which we fill the gap in our lives after a large part of our world has been lost.

Stages of Grief

Just as all those surrounding the patient pass through stages of grief, so does the patient who has learned he is dying. If we understand these stages we can cope more easily with our own feelings and, most important of all, we can better anticipate and meet the needs of the patient.

For the patient the first stage comes immediately after he has been told or has realized that he is dying. He suffers shock and disbelief: "This cannot be happening to me; the diagnosis must be wrong; the doctor does not know everything." It is the same reaction that occurs to parents who refuse to admit that their child is backward or deformed. The shock may be accompanied by physical signs: fainting, pallor, nausea, gastric upsets, rapid pulse or even restlessness and confusion. Sometimes the patient may cry.

This initial reaction is gradually replaced by an awareness of the truth as the reality begins to penetrate the patient's consciousness. He feels sad, hopeless and helpless. He may become angry and blame himself or others. Whatever you do will be wrong. If you want to bath him, he will wish to rest. If you leave him to rest he will say that you are neglecting him. His food will be too hot or too cold and never what he fancies. His medicines and treatments will always be given at the wrong time. He will not want to see his visitors but if they do not come to visit that will also be wrong.

Why is he angry? In effect he is saying: "It is all right for you; you are well, free and able to do what you want; I cannot and will never be able to do so again." He may start to bargain: "If only I can live another six months, I will . . . "; he may become very depressed, withdrawing into himself and not wanting to talk. You may even find him crying quietly. The way you can best help him at this stage is to give him time to grieve. Sit quietly with him and let him talk if he wishes to do so.

This is the point when the patient may derive most help from his spiritual adviser.

The dying patient not only has emotional and physical needs but spiritual needs. Many patients find their religious beliefs all-important in their effort to gain the strength and courage to face their own death with dignity.

The third stage of grief is the acceptance of the inevitable. This final stage brings peace and a sense of wellbeing. The patient will seem more content and may even try and comfort those around him. He may begin to sort out his affairs and a solicitor may be of help.

Your task is to help the patient through these stages and to relieve his loneliness, depression and fears. Most dying patients have three main fears: these are fear of pain, fear of loneliness and fear of the moment of death.

Fear of pain is very common. To help the patient it is important to see that he is kept comfortable and that he receives his medicines on time. The doctor should be told immediately if the prescribed pain-killing drugs are proving inadequate. Fear of loneliness and of dying alone are also very real fears. Most people die when someone is in the room with them, almost as if they hold on to life until they can die in the presence of another human being. Reassure the patient that he will not be left by himself at any time.

Making the Patient Comfortable

As well as helping the patient to cope with his fears and worries, you must also care for his physical wellbeing and comfort. Your aim is to make his last days as happy and relaxed as possible, so that last memories may be pleasant ones.

The dying person has the same physical needs as any other patient. He must be kept clean, comfortable and free from pain. For as long as he is able he should continue to get out of bed, particularly to visit the lavatory or to use the commode. Movement of this kind reduces the risk of pressure sores (see page 29) and gives the patient a little interest and variety.

When the patient becomes too ill to get out of bed his position must be changed every two hours. If he becomes incontinent his skin should be washed and dried carefully and a protective barrier cream applied. An incontinence pad or Kylie sheet may be useful (see page 87). The patient must be helped with his toilet (see pages 40-47) and you should assess the degree of help he requires at any time. Mouth care will be necessary once he is unable to clean his own teeth and if he has dentures you will have to attend to them (see page 46).

The patient's appetite will be failing, so you should offer small appetizing meals of food that he likes. It is essential that he takes adequate fluids: small frequent drinks are more easily tolerated than large ones. Try and avoid a rigid timetable: be prepared to give him a drink or something to eat during the night if he is awake and hungry or thirsty. Vomiting is sometimes troublesome (see page 66). Constipation may also be a problem, which can be avoided by the planned use of suppositories (see page 83).

Many dying patients are not in pain, but those who are need a pain-relieving drug. Such drugs are called analgesics and they range from paracetamol to morphine. The particular drug and the dosage will be determined by the doctor and your task is to ensure that it is given regularly and at the right time. The doctor should be informed if the drugs fail to control the pain or if the patient is no longer comfortable between doses. There is, however, a delicate balance between keeping a patient pain-free and alert. If his last days are to be happy this balance must be achieved.

A Buddhist patient may not wish to have analgesics as Buddhists regard unclouded consciousness as crucial to the finest death. He may, however, be helped by quietness in which to meditate.

If the patient is restless and fails to sleep, other drugs may be prescribed.

The Signs of Approaching Death

The patient grows weaker and sleeps more often. He does not wish to eat or drink. The power of movement and his reflexes are lost; tight bedclothes may bother him so they should be loose and light. You should check frequently to make sure that he has not become incontinent. As his circulation fails, his fingers, toes and nose become blue or mottled. His skin feels cold and clammy and he sweats regardless of the room temperature. This is because the body temperature is rising. Most dying patients are not conscious of being cold; in fact they tend to be restless because they are hot. This fact often needs explaining to those close to the patient.

The patient will probably turn his head towards the light. As sight and hearing fail he only sees what is near and only hears words spoken clearly. For this reason do not draw the curtains or talk in whispers.

As his sensations diminish he no longer feels a light touch, only pressure. This is the time to hold his hand firmly. His breathing will become laboured and noisy. He may become drowsy, go into a very deep sleep or coma, or he may remain quite conscious until the end.

It is difficult to determine how long this period will last, but it is the time when relatives wish to be at the patient's bedside. Seat them comfortably and encourage them to hold the patient's hand and talk quietly to him, whether he is responding or not. Make sure they leave the bedside at intervals to have a meal or a drink and to have a rest. The physical and emotional strain on the relatives during the last days or hours of a patient's life is enormous and it is at this time that the volunteer may be able to give practical help and sympathetic support.

Caring for the Patient after Death

Once breathing has ceased, close the patient's eyelids and leave the relatives with him for a few minutes. Note the time of death. See the family doctor is informed.

When you return to the patient, remove the pillows from the bed, straighten the body gently and lay it flat. If the patient normally wore dentures and they are not in his mouth, clean them and put them in. If there are dressings, colostomy, ileostomy or urinary drainage bags, replace these with clean ones. Cover the patient with a clean sheet and leave him until the undertaker comes. He will attend to everything else. It is a matter of personal preference whether the face is covered or not. Tidy the bedroom and remove all the nursing equipment. If there are flowers, place a vaseful on the bedside table. Once all is tidy the relatives may like to be alone with the patient for a while.

After the undertaker has removed the patient, strip the bed, air the mattress and pillows and open the windows.

Different Religious Beliefs

It is important to remember that certain religions require specific ceremonies at the time of death. Try and find out about them before the patient dies so as to avoid confusion and distress for the relatives.

Jewish and Moslem patients may not be cremated and people who have to touch them after death should wear gloves. Sikhs and Buddhists are cremated and may otherwise be cared for as Christian patients. Hindus like to die at home and often on the floor, to be near mother earth, and this can usually be arranged. They do not require any special care after death.

Helping the Relatives

If the relatives are present when the patient dies, leave them with him for a few moments before leading them gently away. Once the patient has been attended to and the room tidied they may be taken back to the bedside if they wish. Find out if there is anyone they would like telephoned.

When death occurs in a hospital, relatives are usually taken to sister's office and given a cup of tea. When death occurs at home you should stay with them until a friend or another relative has arrived. Initially they may be shocked and unresponsive, however much the death was expected. Presently they may cry or begin to talk, recalling incidents and reliving the past. Sit quietly by them and listen. A silent presence is often very comforting.

Practical Help

A great deal of helpful information is given to the family by the undertaker. He will want to know if any jewellery, such as a wedding ring, is to remain on the patient; if not it should be removed before he leaves.

In hospital a record is made of the patient's valuables and other property. These are then taken to some administrative office in the hospital from which the relatives collect them. A note is kept of any jewellery left on the patient and usually of whether any dentures are in the mouth.

The doctor in charge of the patient certifies death and issues the certificate to the relatives. The death certificate must be taken to the Registrar of Births, Marriages and Deaths. The final funeral arrangements can then be made.

If the doctor has not seen the patient before death or if there are any unusual or suspicious circumstances, he will report the death to the coroner or the appropriate authority. The coroner will then decide whether a certificate can be issued or whether a postmortem examination is necessary. The coroner may conduct an inquest into the death; if he does, the death certificate will be withheld until it has taken place.

Many people have insurance policies especially to cover funeral costs. Most families are entitled to a death grant. It may also help them to know that undertakers vary considerably in their charges. Financial affairs should be dealt with by the family; a family solicitor can be most helpful. The local social security office will be willing to give advice about which forms should be completed for pensions and allowances.

2

USEFUL READING

Introduction:

G Aves, *The Volunteer in Practice*, British Red Cross Society.

R E Bailey, *Volunteers in Hospital*, St John Ambulance Brigade.

P Barefoot and G Cunningham, *Community Services — The Health Workers A-Z*, Faber.

D Gunn, *A Background to Community Care*, British Red Cross Society.

V Henderson, *The Nature of Nursing*, Macmillan, New York.

M Ward, *A Survey of the Health and Social Services*, British Red Cross Society.

P Wilmott, *Consumers Guide to the Social Services*, Penguin Books.

Comfort and Mobility:

Handling the Handicapped (Chapters 4, 5 and 6), Woodhead-Faulkner Ltd in association with the Chartered Society of Physiotherapy.

People in Wheelchairs, British Red Cross Society.

Washing and Bathing:

Handling the Handicapped, Woodhead-Faulkner Ltd in association with the Chartered Society of Physiotherapy.

Clothing:

P Jay, *Help Yourselves* (Chapter 4), Ian Henry Publications.

Catalogue of Clothing, Disabled Living Foundation.

Clothing for the Handicapped Child, Disabled Living Foundation.

Eating and Drinking:

A M Brown, *Practical Nutrition for Nurses*, Heinemann.

P Jay, *Help Yourselves* (Chapter 5), Ian Henry Publications.

Playing Cards, British Diabetic Association.

Elimination:

D Mandelstam, *Incontinence*, Heinemann.

Body Temperature:

R E Bailey and S Carne, *Maternal and Child Health* (Chapters 9 and 10), Textbook of St John Ambulance Association, St Andrew's Ambulance Association and British Red Cross Society.

Communication:

P Jay, *Help Yourselves* (Chapter 10), Ian Henry Publications.

D Ritchie, *Stroke — A Diary of Recovery*, Faber.

Mental Health Guidelines, British Red Cross Society.

Recovery and Rehabilitation:

Plaster of Paris Technique, Smith and Nephew.

Recreational Activities:

G Aves, *The Volunteer in Practice*, British Red Cross Society.

Toys and Ideas for Children when ill, James Galt & Co Ltd (see Useful Addresses).

Learning and Re-learning:

G Aves, *The Volunteer in Practice*, British Red Cross Society.

T Griffiths, *Enjoy Your Retirement*, D & C Newton Abbott.

K M G Keddie, *Action with the Elderly*, Pergamon.

W Loving, *A Lively Retirement*, Queen Anne Press.

Arrangements for Old Age, Consumer Association.

The Patient Who Is Dying:

D Gunn, *Background to Community Care (Bereavement)*, British Red Cross Society.

P Speck, *Loss and Grief in Medicine*, Bailliere Tindall.

When Someone Dies, Consumer Association.

Red Cross Guide to Welfare (Visiting and Counselling; Reactions to Disaster), British Red Cross Society.

USEFUL ADDRESSES

Comfort and Mobility:

Central Council for the Disabled,
25 Mortimer Street, London W1.

Disabled Living Foundation,
364 Kensington High Street, London W14.

Muscular Dystrophy Group,
26 Borough High Street, London SE1.

Rehabilitation Engineering Movement Advisory
Panels, Thomas House North, Millbank, London
SW1P 4PG.

The Royal Association for Disability
and Rehabilitation,
25 Mortimer Street, London W1.

The Spastics Society,
12 Park Crescent, London W1N 4EQ.

Washing and Bathing:

Central Council for the Disabled,
25 Mortimer Street, London W1.

Disabled Living Foundation,
364 Kensington High Street, London W14.

Clothing:

Disabled Living Foundation,
364 Kensington High Street, London W14.

Eating and Drinking:

British Diabetic Association,
10 Queen Anne Street, London W1M 0BD

Disabled Living Foundation,
364 Kensington High Street, London W14.

Marie Curie Memorial Foundation,
124 Sloane Street, London SW1X 9BP

Elimination:

Colostomy Welfare Group
38/39 Eccleston Square, London SW1

Ileostomy Association,
149 Harley Street, London W1.

Breathing:

British Oxygen Company (Medical Gas Orders
and Enquiries), PO Box 17, Medical Works,
Great West Road, Brentford, Middx.

Communication:

British Deaf Association,
38 Victoria Place, Carlisle CA1 1HU

Chest, Heart and Stroke Association,
Tavistock House (North), Tavistock Square,
London WC1.

Mind, 22 Harley Street, London W1M 2ED

Royal National Institute for the Blind,
224 Gt. Portland Street, London W1.

Royal National Institute for the Deaf,
105 Gower Street, London WC1.

Samaritans, 17 Uxbridge Road, Slough, Bucks.

Recreational Activities:

James Galt & Co Ltd.,
30-31 Great Marlborough Street, London W1.

KIDS (Holidays for Socially and Physically
Handicapped Children), 17 Sedlescome Road,
London SW6 1RE

PHAB (Youth Clubs for Physically Handicapped
and Able Bodied), 30 Devonshire Street, London
W1M 2AP.

The British Talking Book Service for the Blind,
Mount Pleasant, Wembley, Middx.

Learning and Re-learning:

Invalid Childrens Aid Association,
126 Buckingham Palace Road, London SW1.

National Society for Mentally Handicapped
Children, Pembridge Hall, 17 Pembridge Square,
London WC2 4EP.

Pre-Retirement Association,
19 Undine Street, Tooting, London SW17.

Remploy, Remploy House,
415 Edgware Road, Cricklewood,
London NW2 6LR.

The Patient Who Is Dying:

Cruse (Help for Widows)
Cruse House, 126 Sheen Road, Richmond,
Surrey.

CONVERSION TABLES

The bold figures in the central column can be read to left or right in each case: for example 35°C equals 95°F, while 35°F equals 2°C.

TEMPERATURE		
Centigrade		Fahrenheit
2	**35**	95
4	**40**	104
7	**45**	113
10	**50**	122
13	**55**	131
16	**60**	140
18	**65**	149
21	**70**	158
24	**75**	167
27	**80**	176
32	**90**	194
38	**100**	212

VOLUME		
Litres		Pints
0.28	**0.50**	0.88
0.43	**0.75**	1.32
0.57	**1**	1.76
0.71	**1.25**	2.20
0.85	**1.50**	2.64
0.99	**1.75**	3.08
1.14	**2**	3.52
1.42	**2.50**	4.40
1.70	**3**	5.28

WEIGHT		
Kilograms		Pounds
0.11	**0.25**	0.55
0.23	**0.50**	1.10
0.45	**1**	2.20
0.68	**1.50**	3.31
0.91	**2**	4.41
2.27	**5**	11.02

LENGTH		
Metres		Yards
0.91	**1**	1.09
1.83	**2**	2.19
2.74	**3**	3.28
3.66	**4**	4.38
4.57	**5**	5.47

INDEX

INDEX

A

Ageing process 134, 150
Analgesics 154
Antacid 66
Anxiety *see Fear*
Aphasia 133
Aseptic technique 116-17
Asthma 126

B

Baby
  bathing 48
  changing napkin 90
  clothing for 56
  dressing 55
  environment for 20-2
  feeding 67-70
  sleep patterns 97
  stools 90
Backrests 31
Bandages
  applying 120, 122
  patterns of 121
  types of 119
Barium X-ray 142
Bath seats 40, 41
Bathing 40-3
  aids to 41
  baby 48
  in bed 43
Bed, adjustable 24
  aids to comfort in 31, 95
  hydraulic 24
  making 24-8
  ripple 29
  stripping 28
  water 29
Bed bath 43
Bed blocks 24
Bed cradle 95, 103
Bedpan 79
Bed rest 24
  positions for 30
Bedwarmers 102
Bicarbonate of soda, solution of 46
Blanket bath *see Bed bath*
Blindness 63, 134, 145
Bottle-feeding 69-70
Breast-feeding 67-8
Breathlessness 127

C

Calories *see Joules*
Carbohydrates 58, 60
Catheter 87
Child
  clothing for 56
  development of 148
  handicapped 148-49
  incontinent 84
  medicines for 76
  sick 98
  See also Convalescence
Cold compress 103
Colic 68
Colostomy 88-9
Comfort in bed 28, 95
Commode 78
Communicable diseases 108-11
  incubation and isolation periods 110-11
Confusion 18, 135
Constipation 82-3
Continental quilt 28, 95
Convalescence 138-39
  activities in 144, 145
  in children 98, 139, 146
Cot 22
  making 24
Coughing 105, 126
  See also Sputum
Cross-infection 106
Cystoscopy 142

D

D & C *see Dilatation and curettage.*
Day centres 65, 141
Day hospitals 140
Deafness 134, 148
Death *see Dying*
Dentures 46
Diabetes 59, 73
Diarrhoea 82
Diet 58-9
  chart 60-1
  and constipation 82-3
  and pressure sores 29
  types of 59
Dilatation and curettage 142
Disabilities *see Handicaps*
Drawsheet 24
  use of 27

Dressing, aids to 51
  a baby 55
  a patient 50
Dressings 118-19
Drops 74
Drugs *see Medicines*
Duvet *see Continental quilt*
Dying 152-55

E

Ear
  ache 107
  drops 74
Eating
  aids to 64
  helping patient with 62-3
Electric blankets 102
Enema 83
  drugs by 73
Eye, care of 45
  drops 74
  stye in 107

F

Faecal incontinence *see Incontinence*
Faeces 82
Fat 60
Fear, in children 98
  of death 152
  of pain 153
  and wakefulness 96, 98
Feeding 62-3
  aids to 64
  baby 67-70
Feminal 86
Fever 103
Fluid
  diet 59
  intake 96
Food 58-63
  See also Diet
Footrests 31
Furniture
  for baby's room 22
  for sickroom 20

G

Gastroscopy 142
Graze 116

H

Hair 47
Handicaps
  clothes for 52-4
  rehabilitation of patients 141, 149
Healing 114
Heartburn 66
Heat, applying 107
Hiccups 126
Hoist 41
Hot spoon bathing 107
Hot water bottle 102
Hydrotherapy 141
Hypothermia 100-1

I

Ileostomy 88
Immunity 112
Immunization 112
Incontinence 84-8
  clothing for 54
  faecal 88
  urinary 84
Incubation period 108, 110-11
Indigestion 66
Infection
  containment of 109, 128
  modes of 108
  in wounds 114
Infectious diseases *see*
  Communicable diseases
Inflammation 106, 114
Inhalation 125
  drugs by 73
Injections 73
  disposable 75
Insomnia *see Wakefulness*
Isolation period 110-11

J

Joules 58

K

Kaolin poultice 107
Kylie bed sheet 87

L

Lavatory, aids in 79
Lice 47
Lifting patient 32-35
  in bath 42
Lymphatic glands 108

M

Meals on Wheels 64, 138
Meconium 90
Medicines 72-6
  care of 75
  categories of 75
  giving 72-4
  giving to children 76
Menstrual fluid 78
Mental illness 135-36
Mineral salts 61
Mouth 46
Mouthwash 46, 103
Moving see Lifting

N

Nails 45
Napkins, baby's 90-2
Nausea 95
  See also Vomiting
Night fear in children see Fear
Nits 47
Noise 20, 96
"Non-touch" technique 117
Nose, blocked 125
Nutrition see Diet

O

Occupational therapy 141
Orthopaedic boards 31
Outpatients 142
Oxygen, giving 128-30

P

Pain
  as cause of wakefulness 97
  suffered by dying patient 153-54
Physiotherapy 141
Pillow, triangular 31
Plaster of paris 142
Plastic pants 91
Pressure areas 29
Protein 60
Pulse, taking 105

Q

Quadruped 37

R

Respiratory rate 105, 127
Retirement 150

S

Sebaceous glands 40
Shaving 44
Sheets, changing 27
Shock 153
Skin 40
    colour 127
Sling 122
Sorbo ring 29
Sores, pressure 29
Speech, difficulties with 133, 135
Sputum 128
Stairlift 37
Sterilizing
    equipment 115
    napkins 91
Stoma 88-9
Stools, in baby 90
    See also Faeces
Stye 107
Suppository 83
    drugs by 73

T

Temperature, body
    in babies 100
    in elderly 101
    high 100, 103
    low 100
    taking 104-5
Tracheostomy 130
Tripod 37

U

Ureter 80
Urethra 80
Urinal 79, 86
Urinary incontinence see Incontinence
Urine 80
    measuring 81
    taking specimen 80
    testing 81

V

Vitamins 60-1
Voluntary aid societies 12-13
Volunteer, role of 11, 14
    relationship with patient 15
    relationship with professionals 16
Vomiting 66

W

Wakefulness
    causes of 94-7
Walking
    aids to 37
    helping with 36
Warmth, aids to 102
Water 61
Water bed 29
Weaning 70
Wheelchairs 38
Wind in babies 68

Z

Zimmer frame 37

NOTES

NOTES

NOTES

NOTES

NOTES

NOTES

NOTES

NOTES

NOTES

NOTES

NOTES

NOTES

176

ACKNOWLEDGMENTS

The text of **Caring for the Sick** was prepared
from material written by Rosemary Bailey, MA,
Dip.Ed., RNT, MTD, Director of Nursing
Education, Hampstead Health District, and a
member of a voluntary organization for over 25
years.

Editor   Sybil del Strother
Designers   Derek Coombes, Ron Pickless

Managing Editor Amy Carroll
Art Director   Debbie MacKinnon

Illustrators
David Ashby
Russell Barnett
John Bishop
Gary Marsh
Jim Robins

Typesetting
Graphicraft Typesetters, Hong Kong

Reproduction
Hong Kong Graphic Arts

Dorling Kindersley would like to thank:
Daphne Crabtree, Paul Fletcher, the Disabled
Living Foundation, volunteers from St. John
Ambulance, London, and the nursing staff of the
Dartford and Grevesham District Health
Authority.